teenage
waistland

teenage
waistland

A Former Fat Kid Weighs in
on Living Large, Losing Weight, and
How Parents Can (and Can't) Help

abby ellin

PUBLICAFFAIRS
new york

Published in the United States by PublicAffairs™,
a member of the Perseus Books Group.

Book design by Jane Raese
Text set in Hoefler

Library of Congress Cataloging-in-Publication Data
Ellin, Abby.
Teenage Waistland : a former fat kid weighs in on living large, losing
weight, and how parents can (and can't) help / Abby Ellin.
p. cm.
ISBN 1-58648-228-9
1. Ellin, Abby 2. Overweight children—United States—Biography.
3. Obesity in children—Treatment. 4. Camps for overweight children.
5. Child rearing.
I. Title.
RJ399.C6E387   2005
362.196'398'0092—dc22
2005041810

FIRST EDITION

2 4 6 8 10 9 7 5 3 1

For my parents
whom I love
and my grandmothers
whom I miss

contents

contents

"The fact is," said Rabbit, "you're stuck."

"It all comes," said Pooh crossly,
"of not having front doors big enough."

"It all comes," said Rabbit sternly,
"of eating too much."

—A. A. Milne, *Winnie-the-Pooh*

acknowledgments

i've wanted to write this book since I was sixteen years old, and I'm still amazed that I finally had the chance. That's largely due to Robert Wilson, my wonderful agent who won't even let me pay for a coffee and always seems to answer my 2 A.M. emails within minutes. His tenacity and enthusiasm led to my genius editor Lisa Kaufman, who transformed a concept into an actual manuscript. Without her vision, patience, wit, insights, and willingness to share her own experiences, I wouldn't be writing this page. Thanks also to Martha Deery, her trusty marketing coordinator, who never seems to leave the office. I've heard horror stories about the publishing industry, but that wasn't my experience at PublicAffairs. Clearly, that's a reflection of Peter Osnos, who runs a terrific company. Nina D'Amario, the creative force behind the book jacket, and Jaime Leifer, my publicity goddess, both deserve awards for putting up with my endless emails and (relatively minor?) obsession about my author photo. Robert Kimzey, Melissa Raymond, and Anais Scott dealt with all the copy-editing and last minute mayhem. Adam J. Sacks, my trusty researcher, could probably find Jimmy Hoffa if he had to. Hats off to you all.

Throughout the years friends have listened to me natter on about fat, either my own or someone else's. They've stuck with me through thick and thin and everything in between. Deepest thanks to: James Alexander Bond, Dave Lewis, Jill Diamond, Pete Ganbarg, Bobby Harrell, Jason Oliver Nixon, Peter Nigrini, Jenny Leigh Thompson, David Wallis, Debra Feldstein, Marybeth Krug, Mark Geiger, Ellen Athena Catsikeas, Ilana Strubel, Julie Slotnik, Tom

acknowledgments

McDonald, Lee Harrington, and Nanette Solow. When we were twelve, Laura Garelick listened to me read my novel-in-progress over the telephone, and actually seemed to enjoy it. Stephanie Winston and Heather Carlucci-Rodriguez, my co-fat farm survivors, are two of my favorite people on the planet. Mary Elizabeth Gifford gave me a place to work. Janet Tashjian, who is always right except when I am, told me I'd never write a book. I think it was reverse psychology, and it worked.

I've been lucky enough to have not one but two mentors, both of whom I consider dear friends: Barbara Adams of the Ithaca College Writing Department and Pamela Painter, the short story writer and a professor in Emerson College's MFA program in creative writing. Barbara encouraged and supported me when I was newly graduated from college, freaked out, with no idea how I was going to make a living as a writer. Pam showed me that the writing life didn't have to be miserable, lonely, and without love.

No one has been more excited about this project than my brother Ray, who's one of the few people I know who lives life on his terms, doing exactly the type of work he loves. Our parents made it possible for us to do what we want to do; the greatest gift any parent can give a child. Other than asking that I not use her real name, my sister gave me carte blanche to write whatever I wanted. I'm grateful for that, as well as to my mother, who didn't censor a word.

Lauren Purcell made wonderful suggestions. Benita Gold corrected my grammar, punctuation, and syntax and (gently) told me when I wasn't being as funny as I thought I was. Hilary Black provided invaluable editorial advice, reading every draft without being afraid to voice her true opinion. Edith Hall Friedheim did not even let one comma go unexamined; she read each page twice and really seemed to care what I had to say. I'm so lucky to have friends like that, as well as editors like Jane Karr, Brent Bowers, and Bob Woletz at the *New York Times,* who have kept me busy over the years. Jim Schachter, my guru, took a chance on a kid, gave her a column, and didn't take it away even when she compared the Roth IRA to Philip Roth.

xii

acknowledgments

So many people took the time to talk with me and share their stories, and I apologize if I inadvertently leave anyone out. I especially want to thank the brave, thoughtful young people who spoke so candidly with me: Emily Isaac, Bryan Tunick, Danielle Rothman, Lindsey Feldman, Benjamin Weill, Josh Gee, Lawrence Capici, Kevin Marema, Kyle Yates, Domnique Gregory, Clara Lay, Shandra Swilling, Alexis Werth Mason, Mitch McConaughey, and Zack Lowe.

The following people opened up their camps, hospitals, homes, schools, and lives to me: Tony Sparber, David Ettenberg, Nancy Lenhart, Ryan Craig and all the students at the Academy of the Sierras, Tammy Cohen, Deborah Frohlinger and all the moms at KIC, Rhonda Capici, Adela Martinez-Regino, Rita Marema, Robert Marema, Terry Weill, Geoffrey Weill, Dr. Julie Germann, Dr. Daniel S. Kirschenbaum and the families in La Rabida's Fit Matters program, Dr. James "Butch" Rosser, Sondra Solovay, Joanne Ikeda, Connie Sobczak, Ellyn Satter, Anne Fletcher, Debby Burgard, Marilyn Wann, Alison Solomon, Alicia Lay, Michelle Gee, Ken Pulos, Beth Swilling, Bonnie Werth, Shawn Lowe and Christina Houghton. My deepest gratitude to you all.

Finally, none of this would be half as exhilarating without Tom Owens. Sometimes the gods do smile.

introduction
fat kid blues

i was ten the first time I stepped on a scale. It was the summer of 1978, and I was visiting my grandmother in Florida.

My family had often spent Christmas vacations in Florida, doing the requisite Disney World/Sea World jaunt, but then, when our happy clan became unhappy and no longer enjoyed being together, I flew down by myself. My grandmother—my mother's mother—and I had a special relationship: she loved my brother and sister, but I was her favorite, or so I liked to believe. She often said I was, but maybe grandparents say this to all their grandchildren, to send them into the world with some semblance of self-worth, however false it may be.

So in the summer of 1978—the year that famed blizzard ravaged the northeast and my sister stopped eating—I went to Florida. I don't know why my folks sent me down; maybe they decided it would be better for me to be out of the house. I didn't mind. I loved traveling, loved being away from home, and I especially loved being with my grandmother.

Grandma's condo was in Margate, a suburb of Fort Lauderdale, and it looked like most of the other buildings in Florida: white-washed walls, rust-colored Spanish-tile roofs, a golf course for a backyard. We did all sorts of things together: shopped at the Bal Harbour mall, swam in the condo pool, ate out at least one meal a day, watched a different movie every week (my favorites were *Heaven Can Wait* and *The Bad News Bears in Breaking Training*). Each morning I woke up in her big bed and she smothered me with kisses. "Good morning, beautiful!" she'd sing, and ask what I wanted for breakfast. Usually, I had a poached egg, toasted bagel, and juicy orange, but sometimes she'd whip up a frothy milkshake (a blended mix of skim milk, ice cubes, and Sweet'N Low). She'd set up a tray for me while I lounged in bed and watched Phil Donahue; later, I'd swim in water heated by the sun. In the afternoon, Grandma and I would go for our daily two-mile walk, past the golf course, past Publix, the supermarket where the old people bought prune juice and cod liver oil. On the way home we'd stop there to weigh ourselves on the gigantic outdoor scale. "Girls have to be thin and beautiful," Grandma would say, always linking the two adjectives together. "The world judges on first appearances."

The routine was the same every day: we'd wait in line behind the old ladies while they handed their packages to their husbands, who seemed tolerant and bored. The women stepped on and off, and then Grandma got on. She didn't look like you'd expect a grandmother to look, soft and round and smelling of gingerbread. No, this Grandma was all sharp angles and points; her make-up and hair carefully arranged, her clothes stylish and neatly pressed. She was interested in modern art, theater, movies, clothes, she took great pride in her appearance, especially her weight. She was skinny, and the needle hovered around 120.

Then it was my turn. I always wanted to take my sandals off, but my grandmother wouldn't let me. She said you never knew what kind of infection you might catch from the person who was on before you. "Don't worry," she said. "We'll subtract a pound for your shoes." She'd peer over my shoulder. "Same as yesterday." Or: "You've lost a pound. Aren't you happy?"

And I was.

Was I ever really fat? Well, no, I suppose. Not technically. As a child I was a gymnast, muscular, firm; my greatest pleasure was going to gymnastics and coming home to a large cheese pizza, oil dripping on my leotard and tights. I loved peppermint stick ice cream, fruit-flavored jelly beans, Duncan Hines chocolate frosting. I loved everything connected with food: reading about it, consuming it, licking bowls. I could devour a box of Ring Dings in an hour and match my father Whopper for Whopper. My food ardor was a family joke of sorts. My mother would name a date and ask me to remember what I'd eaten that day (I usually could), or she would laugh and say if I wasn't careful I'd "blow up like an elephant." Beneath the humor, though, the message was clear: *do not get fat.* During meals, my mother would shoot me dirty looks when I reached for a second helping. But this food-love was never a problem; as a child I ate pleasurably, without guilt. Occasionally, for kicks, I'd step on my mother's little green scale, which sat on the bathroom floor. I'd step on wearing layers of clothes, or a pair of hiking boots, just to see how far the needle could go. The numbers meant nothing to me.

They did to my mother. She weighed herself every morning, immediately after coming back from her daily run around the reservoir (*before* her breakfast of Special K and cappuccino yogurt, lest the outcome be even slightly skewed). The numbers on that scale dictated her mood for the day. If they were higher than usual—even if only by one pound—she'd spend the rest of the morning murmuring about how fat she was, how she had to lose weight, how she couldn't eat more than 1,000 calories. If she and my father had dinner plans, she'd skip breakfast and lunch in preparation for the big meal. This never seemed odd to her. "Everyone does it," she said. "You've got to gear up for an evening out." The next day she'd report, in elaborate detail, what the hostess had served and who had eaten what ("All the fat people had dessert") and how it had taken every ounce of willpower but she had abstained. All the thin people did.

That scale became the focal point of many a lengthy discussion, mainly regarding its precision. Was it accurate? If not, by how many pounds was it off? Was it too heavy or too light? And how could we properly adjust it? When my mother came home from the doctor's office, for example, she'd immediately set our scale to mimic his scale, which must have been exact. Other times my mother set it so it started with three pounds; she was convinced it registered underweight when it began on zero. We all had our little rituals. At the height of my scale-stepping obsession, I'd make sure it sat exactly three linoleum tiles away from the wall, perfectly lined up between squares. It had to be like this each time I weighed myself. Otherwise, there might be inconsistencies.

I can't recall a time when I wasn't conscious that fat was bad. My mother had taped a picture onto the refrigerator of an obese woman rifling through a freezer, a warning of the dangers lurking behind that door. My older sister and I were constantly cautioned by my mother and grandmother never to gain weight. In our minds, getting fat was a terrible tragedy, the worst fate to befall a person. Fat was ugly, undignified, a sign of weakness and failure. But though I was aware of this, I never really worried about it. I could inhale tons of food and burn it off at the gym. Fat, like fatal car crashes or terminal illnesses, was something that happened to other people.

My sister took it all much more seriously than I did. Whenever she ate something fattening she'd turn to my mother, her face taut with panic, and ask, *"Will I get fat? Will I get fat?"* By third grade, she'd dropped sugar altogether and feasted on Original-flavored Cream of Wheat, plain Dannon yogurt, skinless chicken, and mustard-and-Hollywood-bread sandwiches. I was less concerned with my weight, but I do remember calling home from a neighbor's house—I must have been around seven—for permission to sprinkle real sugar, not Sugar Twin, in my tea.

I wanted to be as disciplined as my sister, but I was too much of a hedonist to deprive myself. Only a year and nine months separate us, but we are radically different. People always marveled that we were from the same family, because we were such opposites—"like night and day," they'd say. She was a child prodigy, quiet and studious, an accomplished violinist and math and science whiz who skipped the second grade and starred in an after-school special at age thirteen. I was the amiable one, the sybarite. My sister was intense and focused and methodical; I was a loudmouth, a tomboy, impulsive and headstrong. I couldn't wait to frequent discos and redneck bars and wipe my beer-foam mustache with my shirtsleeve. My father described us this way: "If they were both riding in a car and the driver started speeding, the older one would say, 'Slow down!' and Abby would say, 'Go faster!'"

I admired my sister's restraint with food, but I didn't actively try to emulate it until the sixth grade, right after I returned home from that summer in Florida. I'd watched my grandmother watch her weight and I'd watched my mother watch her weight and I'd watched my sister watch her weight and decided they were right: Girls had to be thin and beautiful. So I began following my sister's regimen, eating plain yogurt for breakfast, half a cheese wedge and banana for lunch, refusing between-meal snacks and bread with dinner. Rather than risk the unnecessary calories found in gum, I chewed the wax that my orthodontist had given me. Thoughts of food assaulted me: I spent my afternoons browsing through cookbooks, tracing my finger along pictures of the desserts I so desperately wanted but would never, ever eat. I weighed myself every morning, checking carefully to see on which number the scale started, and gradually my clothes got looser and my face grew drawn and my ribs and pelvic bones stuck out. People at school noticed, and I loved the recognition I got for not eating. I was unique! I was superior! I was in control! Everyone else ate the cafeteria meals—macaroni with globs of cheese, salads dripping with dressing, sugar-dusted donuts—while I nibbled on my little wedge of cheese, power incarnate.

And then two girls in my class, Carolyn Fisher and Leah Bernstein, went on the Scarsdale Diet, and I was furious. How dare they! *I* was the Dieter; *I* was the special one. True, they were a lot heavier than I was—Leah was downright fat—but I didn't want them to get skinny and be competition. Plus, there was a personal agenda at stake: Leah was mean. She once confessed to taking a nice long snooze while we were on the phone. Instead of hanging up, she simply continued her nap, murmuring *Yeah* and *Uh-huh* at appropriate intervals. Clearly, it was time for revenge.

One afternoon we had a class party to commemorate the end of our section on ancient Egypt. The teacher, Miss Friedman, doled out pretzels and potato chips and Stella D'Oro cookies with a gummy dollop of chocolate in the center. I stared at those cookies, turned one over and over in my hands, but I would not let it touch my lips. But oh! How I wanted Leah to cave in and eat that cookie.

"Come on!" I coaxed, saccharine sweet. "Why deprive yourself? You look great."

"Because I'm on a diet," she said. "I can't have cookies."

"Oh, one cookie won't kill you." I indented the chocolate part of the cookie with my thumb.

"But you're not eating it," she said.

Hmm. She had a point. What to do? "Let's eat them together," I suggested. "At the same time."

She thought for a minute, and then nodded. Slowly, she lifted the cookie to her lips, her eyes never leaving mine: the Sugar Showdown. Everything else in the room faded into the background, except for the sound of the clock ticking on the wall behind me. "Come on!" she urged.

I, of course, had no intention of giving in, but I picked up the treat, brought it up to my lips, and opened wide. Right before my teeth clamped down I snapped my mouth shut, while Leah, the pig, bit in. I watched, gleefully, as she swallowed that cookie in its entirety, hoping the taste of sugar would force her off her diet, making her regain every ounce she'd lost.

"You lied," she said, brushing crumbs off her desk.

I shrugged. "You blew it," I said.

My mother was thrilled with my dietetic zeal—*finally,* I'd seen the light!—just as she'd been pleased with my sister's caloric control. She'd often report to my grandmother how stunning my figure was, how small I'd become. I delighted in this.

Things went along until May 1979, when my other grandmother, my father's mother, visited us and remarked how skinny my sister looked. This grandmother was the antithesis of my other grandmother, more Dr. Ruth than Dr. Atkins. She was tiny—four foot eight (she had to sit on the Yellow Pages when she drove)—wore polyester pants and old lady eyeglasses, shopped at Caldor and Kmart and cared not a whit about Neiman Marcus. She spoke with a softened German accent, and exuded gentleness and goodness, which sounds hokey but it's true. Most of her family had perished in the concentration camps, yet she never seemed angry. Sad, yes, but not angry. She often told stories about Hitler; she forced herself to sit through eight hours of *Shoah,* claiming it was her duty. She valued beauty of spirit over external loveliness—she often quoted *The Picture of Dorian Gray* as a parable—and believed that thinness was important for physical reasons only. (That said, she was very conscious of her height, and whenever she came to visit she would immediately go upstairs and weigh herself on our scale. I guess she'd heard about its amazing accuracy.) Her cupboard was always full of Twinkies and Ring-Dings and Devil Dogs. Whenever I visited we'd create a decadent midnight snack: cake and ice cream, topped off with a thick layer of Cool Whip. She knew my mother would kill her if she found out about it, so we kept it a secret. She'd shrug when I'd mention weight. "Better to be a good person," she'd say, cupping my face in her hands. "Better to be sweet."

My Little Grandma, as I called her, was slightly obsessed with health and constantly clipped articles from *Prevention* and *Reader's Digest* and sent them to her brood. It was she who read a story on anorexia and decided there was something very, very wrong with my sister.

Something *was* wrong, though my parents hadn't seemed to notice. My grandmother insisted my parents take her to the doctor. As a preventive measure, they made me go, too, even though, at four foot eleven, I weighed eighty-three pounds—not too skinny, except I was big-boned and could easily have handled a few extra pounds. The doctor pronounced me underweight—the first and only time that word has ever been applied to me—and I think it was what I'd been waiting to hear all my life. He told my mother I had to stop this craziness or I'd end up like my sister, who must have weighed about seventy pounds.

"I know what's going to happen," I cried, as my mother took me out for my official end-of-diet-meal, a Friendly's hot fudge sundae. "You're going to tell me to eat and I will and then I'll get fat and you'll yell at me to stop."

xxi

My mother sat across from me, watching me spoon ice cream into my mouth and drip chocolate sauce onto the Formica table. She didn't have any ice cream herself, of course. "You might be right," she said.

As it happened, my sister didn't eat, and it took me less than two years to gain twenty-five pounds. I'm not quite sure how the weight-gain began; it built up gradually, tentatively, so slowly I hardly noticed. My interest in food acquired an obsessive quality that, looking back, seems like the early seeds of an addiction. I still don't know if I overate because I had deep-seated problems that could only be calmed by Hostess, or because I genuinely liked sweets. Or maybe problems arose because other people said they were a problem. What are the motivations for *any* obsession? Why do some people pick food, others gambling, others alcohol? The experts, those all-knowing professionals, say that certain addictions are associated with certain classes and ethnicities. I grew up in a white, upper-middle-class Jewish household; maybe it was pre-ordained that my drug of choice would be edible.

After that first hot fudge sundae, I ate like a maniac, like a kid let loose in, well, a candy store. A few months later, in June 1979, I went off to sleepaway camp in Oakland, Maine, and was overwhelmed by the array of unlimited pasta and breads and tins of pudding and cookies and candy and ice cream offered daily in the camp dining hall. I ate whatever I wanted with the same childhood passion; I proudly told everyone I was underweight even though I wasn't anymore. What I remember most about that summer is swapping ghost stories with my bunkmates and slow dancing with Danny Rogers to the Electric Light Orchestra and munching on potato chips and Marathon bars and Charleston Chews and feeling my clothes grow so tight I couldn't button them.

I gained about ten pounds that July, and food became my *raison d'être*. Thoughts of it—acquiring it, paying for it, eating it—consumed me even more than they did during my short-lived pseudo-anorexia phase. At the end of the first session my parents drove up to get me. I wished I could stay for the next four weeks, but they said no, I had to go home for family therapy. Huh?

"But I don't want to do family therapy," I said. All I wanted was to be slow dancing with Danny Rogers, to be pigging out with my friends, to be normal like everyone else. I wanted to jump right out of the car and go to Rummel's for an ice cream cone. (Brand X was their most popular: vanilla mixed with M&M's—very progressive, as this was way before Ben & Jerry's became so popular.)

"Well, your sister's sick and she's got to get better," my mother said. "By the way," she added, "you gained weight."

Over the next year I tried everything in my power to return to underweight-hood: Weight Watchers, Diet Center, Overeaters Anonymous (I went with a friend's mom who was obsessed with being the "perfect wife, perfect mother, perfect daughter, perfect friend." These were not my concerns: I just didn't want to be fat). My mother supported my efforts; she encouraged me and cooked for me and even weighed me, which lasted about two days. I learned how to distinguish four ounces of turkey from six (measure the meat *before* cooking it). I learned how to keep an "honest" record of everything I put in my mouth (if you don't write it down, it doesn't count). I perfected the art of fiction—"Of course I followed the diet. I have no idea why I gained a pound." But my attempts were fruitless; I could never diet for more than a day. Like Oscar Wilde, I could resist everything but temptation . . . and peanut butter cups. And M&M's. And ice cream. And pizza. I loved food. I just hated being bigger than everyone else.

Not surprisingly, food stopped being a source of pleasure and became, instead, the enemy. My body will never be as slight as Kate Moss's (will anyone's?), but as an adolescent I yearned for nothing more than matchstick legs and pelvic bones as sharp as steak knives. I desperately wanted to be thin again, but I resented the sacrifice. One of my few delights was eating—why deny myself? (After the initial horror of 9/11 dimmed, my philosophy was, "Well, if the terrorists are going to get us, we might as well eat . . .")

A little over a year later my Florida grandmother came to visit for the Jewish New Year. I hadn't seen her in nearly twelve months. As usual, she looked wonderful, her nails newly manicured, her clothes freshly pressed. She kissed me hesitantly, her hands kneading the strange new flesh on my shoulders and back. She was horrified.

Later, I overheard her telling my mother that I'd gotten "tremendous." At dinner, I reached for a second slice of kugel, and my grandmother slapped my hands away. "You don't need another," she said. "How can you let yourself go like this? You've got such a gorgeous face—don't you want boys to like you? Don't you care what people think when they see you?"

"Ma, don't," my mother said, dipping an apple sliver into a bowl of honey.

"You've got to get hold of yourself," Grandma continued. "You need to lose fifteen pounds or else you can't come to Florida this Christmas."

"But why?" I said, tears burning my eyes. "Who cares what I weigh?"

"Because the world judges on first appearances," Grandma snapped. "Don't argue with me. It's my home and I don't want you there unless you look the way you're supposed to." As further incentive, she told me she'd buy me a whole new wardrobe if I lost weight.

"But it's a big state," I stammered, trying to joke. "I can fit."

"No," she said, and I knew she meant it. I was devastated. This was the worst thing she could possibly have done. I loved Christmas in Florida, and looked forward to it all year long. I'd made a lot of good friends there, the grandchildren of the other old people who lived in my grandmother's condo complex, good friends I only saw one week a year. It was where I had my first crush, on a boy named Brad from Marlboro, New Jersey, and, thanks to a hearty game of Truth or Dare, my first kiss. It's the place I perfected Ping-Pong and shuffleboard, where I learned to smoke cigarettes and drink Riunite and, of course, step on scales.

I'm sure my grandmother meant well, and was only doing what she thought was helpful. And what teenager wouldn't want free rein in Bloomingdales and Burdines? But it didn't seem to be enough.

Over the next few months she clipped diets from magazines and mailed them to me. Her favorite was the Weigh of Life, a program that incorporated fruits, vegetables, and lots of protein into a daily regimen. Her passion was militant. "You really have to look at this as a way of life," Grandma said over the telephone. "You've got to think of fattening foods as poison—things that will kill you if you eat them."

My mother tried to help. She cooked low-fat, low-calorie meals, weighed and measured everything on my plate. She labeled the food in the refrigerator. Healthy stuff had my name taped on it, the more fattening stuff was for my father, brother, or "company." (My sister was in charge of her own meals, such as they were.) I tried to be good, tried to eat salads without dressing and only one slice of pizza. And yet I constantly wondered why I was depriving myself. Would lead roles come my way if I got thin? Would the National Merit Scholarship people call me? Would guys pound on my door until it caved in? Part of me doubted this, while another part *did* believe my life would magically transform itself once I knocked off ten pounds. And so I kept trying, but that would only last a few days. Then my body would feel weak and sluggish and my thoughts would focus on what I wanted to eat and what I couldn't eat and why I couldn't eat it. Sometimes the hunger was so bad I'd rummage through my mother's purse and pluck out a ten- or twenty-dollar bill. I'd stuff it into my pocket and head to the nearest supermarket, buying boxes of Twinkies and bags of jelly beans. I buried them in my middle drawer, beneath my bras and collection of foreign currency, locking my bedroom door while I ate.

I wasn't the only one who hid food. Every so often I'd open a cabinet, a storage bin, and find chocolate or donut holes stuffed into brown paper bags. Once I even discovered an apple pie in the trunk of mother's Cadillac. I'd slip the goodies inside my shirt and sneak upstairs to my room. The next day I'd shove the wrappers in my knapsack and toss them into a garbage can at school. One day I came home from school to find my mother waiting for me, an empty box of Devil Dogs in hand. "Where the hell did this go?"

I shrugged and flipped my palms, looked her straight in the eye. "How would I know? I didn't even know you had that," I lied. "Ask your other children."

My mother laughed sadly. "Ray's too young, and you know your sister wouldn't eat that. She won't eat anything."

That was true. While I was getting bigger, my sister was still wasting away, her bones sticking out like wire hangers, her belt cinched twice around her waist. She'd lock herself in her room for hours, doing sit-ups and leg lifts. She'd actually removed the mattress from her canopy bed, installed a weight set where the bed used to be, and slept on the floor. Why my parents let her do this still puzzles me. I guess it was easier to give in than to fight.

At mealtimes my mother's eyes would dart between my plate, which was full, and my sister's, which was organized like a closet: chicken in one compartment, peas in another, mashed potatoes in a third. She chopped her food into sixteenths, chewed each piece twenty times, careful not to let her fork touch her lips. She still exercised daily, running five, six times around the reservoir. We had long ago stopped family therapy and she was seeing her own counselor, but I didn't think it was doing much good.

"Where did you hide that?" I asked, trapping her. "*Why* did you hide that?"

My mother looked at me and then at the empty box of Devil Dogs, back and forth, back and forth, as if the answer lay in the space between. "Because you're fat," she said finally. "I love you, but you're fat."

I jerked backwards, as if she had punched me in the gut. "Then how can you love me?"

I did not go to Florida that Christmas.

» «

xxvi

My mother doesn't especially like to talk about all this; it took place well over twenty years ago, and the memories simply aren't as potent for her as they are for me. (My sister and I *never* go there.) She has phased out a lot of specifics from that time. Still, I remember her calling up another mother whose daughter was anorexic, and I remember her crying into the phone.

"I felt terrible that my child was sick," she told me recently. "I felt helpless that nobody seemed to be able to help her no matter what we tried."

Did she worry about me? And if not, why did she give me so much grief for being overweight? "I didn't worry that you'd get sick because you were fat, but I worried that you would suffer the consequences of a society that viewed slenderness as desirable," she said.

"So how come you told me one thing in one breath—that I had to be thin—and then in another breath told *her* that she was too skinny?" I asked. "Rather hypocritical, don't you think?"

She was silent for a few minutes. Finally, she repeated the same mantra she uses whenever I question her parenting: "I didn't know what to do. I did the best I could."

The best I could. The best I could. At the time, that wasn't enough, but now that I'm older I get it. I understand her frustration, and her inability to do the "right" thing. Is there *ever* a right thing when it comes to parenting?

I'm betting this sounds familiar to you, too, especially if you are or have ever been a fat kid. If you're the parent of one you might see yourself in my mother, faced with a child who has some kind of weight problem, and not knowing what to do. And so you try anything and everything: modeling calorie-conscious behavior; storing healthy food in the cupboard; supporting his or her efforts to diet and exercise; trying behavior modification and setting up rewards for success. But you mainly succeed in making your kid feel bad, ugly, angry, guilty, and miserable.

Only now, with friends stumbling through parenthood, do I really get what my own folks had to deal with and how absolutely flummoxed they were. You never know how your kid is going to turn out, but I doubt my parents expected their two daughters to spend their adolescences fixated on weight. It's fascinating, if you think about it: My sister and I both received the same messages about fat, but we handled them so differently. What made me internalize them one way and her go the other route? What made her shun food, and me run toward it? And what the hell should my parents have done for either of us? It must have been heartbreaking for them, desperately wanting to help their kids while being utterly incapable.

Not that I let them off the hook completely. I spent years condemning my folks (well, mostly my mother) for even making food an issue in the house. If my mother had her own issues under wraps, I believed, my sister and I would never have had to suffer. I still believe this is true, but I don't resent my mother—or even my grandmother—anymore. Now that I'm older, I feel bad for them, for all of us. It's hard enough just to survive on this planet; most people are simply doing the best they can. Yes, some people absolutely have no business reproducing. But the average person—my own parents, you—truly wants what's best for their kids. If they only knew what that was, or how to bring it about, things would be a lot easier.

» «

I'm not a fat kid anymore, but I've remained almost fanatically interested in the issues that arise around food, weight, and families. I've talked to hundreds of fat kids and former fat kids; I've talked to the parents of fat kids and dozens of experts and professionals who treat fat kids. And now that childhood obesity has been deemed a cultural crisis there are plenty of books and magazine articles being published on these subjects, which I read religiously. I'm always curious to see whether anyone has figured out yet how to deal with weight issues better than my family dealt with mine. The answer, not surprisingly, is a resounding *no*. Most of the books preach a fitness and nutrition philosophy, which is pretty much the same type of message my mother and grandmother tried unsuccessfully to impart to me. But the experts are oddly mute when it comes to the subject of how exactly to implement their wisdom and what to do when your kid sabotages or rebels against or simply isn't interested in the suggestions; or tries to get thin but tires of the healthy new regime after their weeks of effort yield few tangible results; or complains of being hungry and miserable; or hates you thoroughly for even mentioning the subject of weight, thereby making his or her miserable existence even *more* miserable. What these books do seem to take for granted, though, is that parents have got to do something, because your kid's weight is clearly your problem.

Michael Fumento, author of the book *Fat of the Land* (Viking, 1997), says out loud in a 1997 interview in *Salon* what many people seem to think: "Kids live basically in a dictatorship while they are in their parents' home. When a kid is grossly fat, that is the parents' fault."

Many parents do feel responsible—even when they've been trying for years to help their kids lose weight. "Your anxiety is that you have ruined the child forever or that they will be taken away from you because you've made them fat," says Lisa Williams, the mother of fourteen-year-old Emily, who weighs 250 pounds. Williams has been shuttling her daughter to nutritionists, psychologists, endocrinologists, support group meetings, and weight-loss camps for the last five years. "I'm worried about seeing her alienated, alone, unloved, made fun of, deprived of opportunities. I probably would calm down a great deal if Emily grows up and finds love and a wonderful partner and actually likes what she does and is basically happy, even if she never gets as thin as she should be. But when I see her using food in a compulsive way to escape feelings and to pad herself against the horrors of life, it's heartbreaking."

Williams might find it reassuring to know that even so-called experts have difficulty when it comes to their own kids and food. (One-time *Pumping Iron* guru Arnold Schwarzenegger's daughter has extra meat on her bones, though his wife seems to be dissolving before our eyes.) Anne M. Fletcher is a registered dietician and the author of the terrific *Thin for Life* (Houghton Mifflin, 2003), as well as a forthcoming book on teens who have successfully lost weight. She has won a number of awards and knows more about the subject of dieting and healthy eating (and sobriety, for that matter) than almost anyone I know—and yet her oldest son, who is now twenty-one, was sixty pounds heavier as a teenager. "It was very difficult and embarrassing," she admits. "I'm supposed to be this expert and here's my fat kid." Eventually he did lose weight, but it took time. "He needed to find his own solution," she says.

Most kids are not especially thrilled with their parents' efforts to help them deal with their weight. "Adults think they know more about how I feel than I do," says thirteen-year-old Caitlin Armstrong, who weighs 185 pounds. "They really don't know what's going on inside an overweight child's head."

"One time I said something mean to my father—I don't remember what—and he said to me, 'Well, at least I don't hide candy in my sock drawer,'" recalls Danielle Webber, thirteen, who recently lost twenty pounds. "That really hurt. I could not believe my father said that to me. I stood up and walked away from the kitchen table."

(My friend Benita Gold, who was slightly heavy as an adolescent, still remembers the motivational record her mother handed her when Benita turned twelve, entitled, *Mary Ann Mobley Wants to Have a Heart-to-Heart Talk with You, Chubby.* Apparently the former Miss America had had a weight problem, conquered it, and wanted to impart her wisdom.)

"Most people don't get it," says Bryan Morris, sixteen, who once weighed 220 pounds and is now about 190. "Obesity is not a disease, it's more of a disorder or an addiction. And yet people don't deal with it with enough sensitivity. The more aware the world is of problems—not just obesity—the worse we deal with them. For example, if we tell parents 'Hey, watch out—obesity is a huge problem and make sure it doesn't happen to your kid,' parents are going to strike back. But when you do whatever you can to prevent a problem, at the same time you're doing your best to cause it." In other words, adolescent logic dictates that the more parents freak out about their children's weight and the more they bug them about it, the more their kids are going to want to rebel.

If kids react that way to their parents' concern, imagine how they respond to the messages they get from the world. Fat hysteria has swept the nation, with talk of taxes on foods that are high in sugar and fat, and lawsuits against fast food companies. You can't go anywhere without hearing that childhood obesity is near epic proportions, an epidemic (as if fat could be transmitted from one person to the other through the sheer force of our cultural anxiety), a national health risk, a code orange of fat young people. Nearly every health organization and government agency from the American Cancer Society to the U.S. Department of Agriculture has issued guidelines for preventing obesity, mostly through diet and exercise. The mission of the new millennium seems clear: *Help the fat kids, help the fat kids!*

And why not? There are big bucks to be made from it. The diet industry, after all, is a $46.3 billion business; in 2003, Weight Watchers had revenues of $1 billion. By the end of 2003, Jenny Craig, with 680 centers nationwide, had $280 million in sales. Thanks to the late Dr. Atkins and his diet revolution, the world is now filled with legions of anti-carb acolytes. In January 2004, representatives from 450 companies—including Kraft, ConAgra, and Wal-Mart—even gathered for a two-day Low Carb Summit, God help us, to discuss those Weapons of Mass Carbohydration. Of course they did. Why shouldn't they get a piece of the low-carb pie, too?

Indeed, there are so many weight-loss theories out there, and so many approaches and diets, and so many experts who claim to have The Answer—many of whom, like the oft-quoted Kelly D. Brownell, director of the Yale Center for Eating and Weight Disorders and the coauthor of *Food Fight* (McGraw-Hill, 2003), have not conquered their own weight demons—that it's hard to know what to believe or whom to trust. Everyone has an opinion and an agenda that's often expressed with a smug, superior, holier-than-thou attitude—without saying anything enlightening or new.

Here, to spare you years of research and reading (in the unlikely event that you haven't been doing it already), is a handy summary of all this opinion: Kids are too fat, and it's a terrible, terrible problem. Kids should expend more calories than they take in and eat low-fat high-fiber foods and/or low-carb foods. Parents should help them lose weight. You should also change your whole family's lifestyle. Fast food: bad! The Internet: horrendous! Society should change, and parents should spearhead the effort. You can do it! Fat is disgusting and a sign of weakness and moral failure. Good-bye and good luck!

The trouble is, earnest iterations of good nutrition and physical fitness advice, and critiques of fast food, food marketing, unhealthy school lunches, and TV, don't in and of themselves work.

Emily Williams has been grappling with her weight since she was eight, has spent three summers at weight-loss camps, and is on a first-name basis with most diet doctors in Manhattan. She speaks for just about every overweight person everywhere when she says, "I know what I need to do. I could probably write the book on it. I just can't do it."

While there are certainly plenty of parents who are ignorant about basic nutrition, lots are already well versed in fruits and veggies and skim-milk products. Most of you reading this book—and probably most of your kids—know how to lose weight, at least in theory. Chances are you've bought a food scale and a tape measure and been mired in diet culture for years. If you're like the majority of Americans, you've earned your diet wings yourself. It's common sense, really: expend more than you take in. But knowing what to do and actually doing it—at any age—are two entirely different animals, for our culture as a whole and for the individuals in it. (Ever tried to stop drinking or smoking? Not fun. Nor easy.)

Sure, parents are aware that their kids should get active, but what if your kid's (or your!) idea of exercise is lifting the spoon to his mouth? A post-dinner stroll would be hell. Shuttling your kids outside to play is a lovely thought—but how many families live in truly bucolic and safe suburban settings where other kids are getting their heart rates up in the backyards while all the stay-at-home moms keep a watchful eye? And let's be real: There are not a whole lot of openings on the track team for a fat kid (as if the thought of gasping and panting and sweating one's way to last place were remotely appealing). Gym class can be torturous even if you're a normal size. And private gyms? Kids under fourteen aren't really allowed in, and those who are old enough probably don't want to be the sole heavy amid the hard bodies.

Plus, once kids begin to operate outside the bounds of complete parental control—to spend time at school, for example, or to go on playdates, or to morph into adolescents—they, not you, are in charge of their own choices. If your kid is a freethinker or has authority problems—a condition common among the fifteen-year-old set—the rebellion against your hopes and expectations for them will be that much more pronounced.

Look, losing weight is *hard.* Dieting makes you cranky and edgy and gloomy and moody, and who wants to go without? We are a nation of attention-deficit-afflicted hedonists; we want to have our cake, scarf it down, and stay thin. Who wants to expend the time and effort when you might not see results for weeks, months, or even years? Most weight-loss groups, like Weight Watchers, recommend a one- to two-pound loss a week. If you've got, say, a hundred pounds to lose, that's about a year before your weight loss will even be noticeable—and after all that effort, you'll still be big. Now try convincing your kid to try it.

(Ironically, in 2002 Weight Watchers stopped allowing children under ten to attend meetings; kids eleven to seventeen need a physician's note to participate. "Adult programs don't work for kids," says Karen Miller-Kovach, MS, RD, chief scientific officer at Weight Watchers International, in Woodbury, New York. A few years ago, Miller-Kovach and her colleagues reviewed all the literature on childhood obesity and found that there really hadn't been a lot of work done in the field. "It's an area of emerging science, and we're finding that a lot of things don't seem to work," says Miller-Kovach, who is in the midst of developing a Weight Watchers program for children and adolescents.)

Few if any of the thousands of books and articles written on this subject address these facts. To them, weight loss is a technical issue rather than the enormously time-consuming, lifelong, life-changing struggle that it is, involving complex and complicated variables: emotions, addiction, genetics, psychological and medical issues, self-esteem, motivation, shame, depression, willpower, peer pressure, family dynamics, parental relationships, sexual identity, pleasure, deprivation, and our culture's strong signals about appearance and self-worth. One size does not fit all when it comes to weight loss, and the better we understand that, the more likely we are to arrive at real solutions for kids and a more sophisticated understanding of the problem itself.

Before I go any further, a few admissions: I am not a parent, and have never been one. I've never even been married. But I am a former fat kid. I spent six years at various weight-loss camps around the U.S.: two as a camper, four as a counselor. Like so many women—and yes, men—I have devoted an enormous amount of brain space to calories and carbohydrates and the size of my thighs. As an adolescent I stepped on the scale four, five, six times a day, rocking back and forth, hoping the needle would move farther to the left, panicking if I gained a pound. I often used food as a drug, and my weight as a barometer for success and well-being. I lived life in the future tense: *I will be happy when I'm thin. I will be famous when I'm thin. I will fall in love when I'm thin.*

Technically, I was never obese. At most I was twenty-five pounds heavier than I should have been—thirty if you consider that at five foot two and three-quarters I'm "supposed" to weigh 110. But those extra pounds ruled my life, as well as the lives of my family, who genuinely seemed to dislike me when I was "chunky." Those twenty-five pounds had an enormous impact on my self-esteem; my self-worth depended on the numbers on the scale, and yet nothing I tried—and nothing my mother and grandmother tried—inspired me to stop eating. My father, for his part, tried to reason with me, telling me that my health was at risk. Actually, it wasn't. I was very healthy, no diabetes or heart problems on the horizon. And though health was supposedly the most important reason for my losing weight, he was not above making less high-minded comments. Once, playing tennis with him, I removed my eyeglasses just as two guys walked onto the court next to us. "That's the wrong thing to lose," my dad said. Nice.

The badgering got so bad that I finally stopped eating with my family. I'd sneak food into my bedroom—hoard it, actually—and chow down by myself, as your own kids probably do. Eventually, I went to one weight-loss camp and then another and then another and lost weight and gained weight and lost it again over the course of a decade. I'm not kidding when I say that keeping my weight off has been one of my greatest, and most challenging, efforts. It's a daily struggle, perched smack in the center of my brain. On many levels, it governs my life. (I have always longed to join the Peace Corps, for example, but I worry: *Where can I get a Lean Cuisine in the Amazon? Can you burn calories teaching English in Tonga?*)

I've also spent years trying to figure out how parents should cope with their "nutritionally challenged" child and what our culture could do but doesn't (besides elevating the terror alert on weight). I've devoted a lot of time and energy over the years—perhaps too much—wondering what, if anything, my own parents should have done differently, and whether it would have even worked, or been enough. Who would I be today if they had left me alone? Would I have ballooned to 300 pounds, or would my body have wound its way back to its natural set point? Would I have grown into a pillar of emotional well-being without any existential crises, or would I have become depressed and suicidal? Should my folks have tried different tactics, or just left me to my own devices and learned to mask the disgust on their faces when they saw me? Yes, it would have been nice if they accepted me as I was—and since I wasn't, technically, all that big, they could have. On the other hand, the world is brutal and unforgiving. Our appearance is endlessly appraised, as my grandmother was well aware. It affects our love life, work life, and self-esteem. Is it not, then, irresponsible to ignore this fact and pretend it doesn't exist?

We really do have a growing weight problem. According to the latest federal figures, the percentage of youngsters age six to eleven who are overweight has tripled since the 1960s. As many as one in five kids is overweight or obese, and doctors are seeing children as young as three who weigh in at 120 (and 400-, 500-, and even 600-pound teenagers). And obesity is not just an aesthetic issue: Overweight children are more than twice as likely to have high blood pressure or heart disease as children of normal weight. They're also susceptible to Type 2, or non-insulin-dependent, diabetes, which puts them at risk for blindness, nerve damage, kidney failure, and cardiovascular and adult heart disease.

But few parents—black, white, or Hispanic, moneyed or not, well-educated or less so—seem to know what they're doing when it comes to food, kids, and weight. Sure, sometimes it's because they have no clue about the proper feeding of another being, which is what all the current books and articles seek to remedy. But there are other reasons, too, which aren't identified or addressed. Some parents have their own struggles with food and weight. Some waver between strategies for helping their kids, and founder among the mixed messages. Some feel reluctant to structure their family's whole life around weight loss—which is what appears to be required. Others tire of trying to force a resistant kid to do something he or she doesn't want to do, creating more frustration and unhappiness in the process, upsetting and alienating their child rather than helping them. For these parents, knowing what they should do and what should happen doesn't help them with the fundamental issue: how to maintain enough energy and motivation to keep inspiring a kid who loves eating more than she loves doing the hard work necessary to lose weight.

Many cultural and social critics like Greg Critser, the author of *Fat Land* (Mariner Books, 2004), seem to think that each one of us needs to be a lot more ashamed and appalled about the situation, that our problem is that we're just not disgusted enough with ourselves (and, by extension, our kids). We should stop enabling fat kids by, for example, allowing retail chains like Torrid to design fashionable clothing to fit them. If the kids looked even uglier, this line of thinking seems to suggest, they'd be more motivated to get thin.

He's wrong. How much worse could kids possibly feel? Fat kids are, more often than not, treated horribly by their peers and their parents—which is almost more damaging, I believe, than their physical struggles. A study by the University of Michigan and the University of Medicine and Dentistry of New Jersey surveyed 17,500 adolescents and found that the overweight kids had fewer friends than normal-weight kids. In 2003, University of Minnesota researchers interviewed 4,746 kids in grades seven to twelve and found that overweight teens are more likely to be depressed and more suicidal than their skinnier peers. Why? Because of all the teasing, said study author Marla Eisenberg.

Overweight adolescents are also more apt than normal-weight children to be victims and perpetrators of bullying, a study in the May 2004 edition of *Pediatrics* reported: the oppressed becoming the oppressor. And then there's the oft-quoted study in which obese kids rated their quality of life with lower scores than young cancer patients on chemotherapy. If that's not enough, one report found that 11 percent of all people would abort their child if they knew it was genetically predisposed toward fat.

I don't know why any of this is especially shocking. Ask any fat kid what his life is like and he'll tell you how awful it is, how everyone, from peers to teachers to parents, views him as defective (if he's viewed at all—the most invisible people are often the most visible). How he'd rather stay at home with a bucket of fried chicken than venture into the real world. How he'd rather die than face his schoolmates.

In March 1995, *ABC-20/20* devoted an entire segment to growing up fat. At one point, reporter John Stossel asked a group of five-year-olds who they would rather have as a friend, a stupid kid or a fat kid.

"Stupid," the kids replied.

"Which would you rather be?" Stossel asked. "Ugly or fat?"

"Ugly!"

"If you had to live your life without one arm or fat, which would you pick?"

"One arm! One arm!"

Twelve-year-old Andrea Thompson says she "hates" herself because she weighs 230 pounds. "Sometimes I wish I could just end it once and for all," she says. "I feel worthless and stupid; sometimes there's nothing I hate more than waking up every day and realizing I'm the same person."

"It is really amazing the psychological effects being even slightly overweight can have," says Laura O'Brien, fifteen, and 190 pounds. "It changes your perspective on everything and everybody. When you meet someone, one of the first things you think is about how your body compares to theirs. I have one friend who's slightly more overweight than I am, and she's so uncomfortable with it that she lies about weight and size, when it's obvious that she's not what she claims."

It's hardly surprising that by age nine children have developed an active dislike of fat bodies—or that, as a San Francisco study of 500 girls reports, almost half of the nine-year-olds were already dieting. By age twelve, it was up to 80 percent.

For a fat kid, the loneliness and alienation is never ending. As most of us know—whether we've experienced it firsthand, watched others grapple with it, or been perpetrators ourselves—fat is the last acceptable form of discrimination. You can't comment on race, religion, gender, sexual preference, or height, but a fat person is fair game.

There's a hierarchy to polite conversation: sex, money, fat. That is: Most people freely talk about their sex lives; some people discuss their finances; but few disclose their weight or true eating habits. Doctors—many of whom, let it be noted, are not ideal physical specimens—often discriminate against their fat patients.

Fat prejudice is also ageless. Diane Russo, a New York public relations executive who is well into her sixties, says with only mild embarrassment: "I have no fat friends; I'm too shallow. I know it's terrible, but that's how I am."

Even the media, which is allegedly trying to raise awareness about the issue, is hypocritical. About a year ago I met a *National Geographic* photographer who was snapping pictures for a cover story on obesity. She was worried about the photos, though; when she showed her editor the first batch, the editor had turned away in horror.

"Why is everyone so fat?" she asked, aghast.

"Um, because it's a story about fat people . . . ?" the photographer said.

"Yes, but how can I sell magazines with fat people in them?" the editor said. She was completely serious. The issue subsequently ran in August 2004. The cover features a naked torso with rolls of fat; it looks like an erotic photo of the tundra. There is not one photograph of a fat person inside the magazine, although some do appear on the Web site.

On October 27, 2003, *ABC News* aired a special called "Fat Like Me: How to Win the Weight War." The producers stuffed a fifteen-year-old girl named Ali Schmidt into a fat suit, causing her weight to balloon to 230 pounds (in real life she's five foot six and 126 pounds). They filmed her attending classes at a school where no one knew her. She was given a tiny camera that she placed in her backpack to record her fellow students' reactions. Not surprisingly, she was assaulted with all sorts of barbs: Boys were rude to her face; the girls ignored her. (Her two science-lab partners made eye contact only once). "I told myself it was a costume," Schmidt told *People* magazine, "but I felt miserable."

Lucky for her she was able to shed her girth and enjoy every fat kid's dream: She returned to school the next day at her normal weight and blew the other kids' minds. Did the students learn a lesson? Not really. "It was funny," said a boy who had laughed at Schmidt when her rear end bumped the lunch tray and knocked it over.

Nor did it impress a lot of the kids who have been on the receiving end of those taunts. Bryan Morris, who still struggles with his weight, says, "It annoyed the hell out of me to see them put that girl in a fat suit. She at least had the comfort of knowing that she was going to get out of it. If I'm going to watch a girl cry about being fat, she better be fat."

Clearly, if shame were motivational, a lot of fat kids would be thin by now.

When the shame-ourselves-into-action approach doesn't work, some parents turn to the opposite theory: that, in the words of fat-acceptance guru Paul Campos, obesity is a myth; that self-acceptance is more important than size; that loving yourself no matter how heavy you are and concentrating on cultivating as healthy a lifestyle as possible, rather than on weight loss per se, is the goal. But even assuming that Campos is right when he says that the relationship between obesity and health isn't as clear-cut as diet-industry-funded research studies seem to indicate, in the world in which we live, and in which kids become adults, self-acceptance would be as big and impossible a job as . . . well, weight loss. (Campos, it should be noted, whittled his own body down from 210 to 160 pounds—which he both proudly and ashamedly admits in the last chapter of his book. Even he, an academic who is deeply aware of how complicated this all is, is not free from fat-induced self-loathing.)

In an ideal universe, society *would* change. Fat kids wouldn't be ridiculed, soda machines would be used as art projects, school lunches would be tasty and nutritious, television sets across the country would somehow melt into the ether, the Information Superhighway would come to a screeching halt, and the good folks at Duncan Hines, Nestlé, and Hostess would stop producing junk (albeit tasty junk). But while we're waiting for this to happen, parents need some kind of help. The question is, What?

In the meantime, what should you and your kids do in the world we live in today, with all of its temptations and triggers? What, if anything, can you say to kids that they will hear? What can you do if your kid isn't sufficiently motivated to lose weight? Do you send her to fat camp? Do you push him onto the treadmill, or staple his stomach? Do you sue Entenmann's? What, in terms of treatment methods, actually works? Willpower or surrender? Diets or gradual lifestyle changes? Strict supervision or faith in your child's ability to change on her own? Do you annoy your slightly pudgy kid until she either starves herself or plows through everything in the house and becomes twice as heavy? Do you let it go because a few extra pounds don't matter—until he develops Type 2 diabetes or sleep apnea and the world sees you as a colossal parental disaster? Conversely, is it irresponsible if you don't harass him and he blows up to a size 25? And then what do you do to clear your name?

Keep in mind that this is not a book filled with suggestions to keep fresh veggies in a Ziploc bag and to go for walks as a beaming cardiovascularly healthy family unit. It's about exploring the human side of being a fat kid in a thin-obsessed world, about figuring out how to achieve something incredibly difficult in an environment that sets you up for failure. It is a book for all the fat kids who have tried it all, or who can't bring themselves to try; who have been judged and ridiculed and blamed. It's for all the parents who have overdosed on grilled skinless chicken breasts and diet Jell-O for their children's sake with no tangible success. It's for you, who would do anything for your overweight child but simply don't know the best course.

What works? Let's find out.

I

ho hos in paradise

my stomach rumbles beneath the sheets, from hunger or
nerves or both, and I awaken with a jolt. Normally, I would
rather lounge in my bunk bed until noon, but today's different. It's
weigh-in day at Camp Colang, a Weight Watchers camp in the
Pocono Mountains. This is what I've been working toward all week,
and the sooner I wake up, the sooner I find out if my efforts have
paid off. The tension is as thick as a chocolate milkshake. It is the
summer of 1984, and I am sixteen years old.

Every Sunday after breakfast—it's the same every week: scrambled egg and minibagel ("egglet and bagelet"), a pat of margarine, a
four-ounce glass of OJ, and a cup of skim milk—we trudge the hundred yards to the triangular-shaped building that houses the two
doctor's scales. We strip down to our bathing suits or T-shirts, tossing our sweatshirts and jeans aside. Health regulations apply; everyone must wear shoes. We slip on rubber thongs or Ked sneakers
—no one wants to add unnecessary pounds.

These weekly weigh-ins are rituals, structure that we fat people
need. As camp director Tony Sparber often tells us, we're heavy because we have no discipline; we need some kind of order in our
lives. The scale is our god, the Weight Watchers food program our
Bible, "Skinny arms!" our mantra.

Before stepping into the closed-off room where the scales are
(privacy is of utmost importance), a counselor hands out index
cards with our vital statistics, updated each week: the amount of

weight we've lost, and the measurements of our arms, legs, waist, thighs, calves, and bust. My friend Stephanie Winston glances at her card. "If I don't lose at least two pounds I'll die!" she moans. I nod sympathetically. Last week she only lost half a pound—*half a pound*—and she was all set to go home to Manhattan, where she could at least have her own room and a hot shower. This is her fourth year at camp, and she's promised herself it's her last, as she does every summer.

We wait in line until one of the friendly food advisors motions me into the room. "Step on the scale," she says, and slides the metal bar to the number it was the previous week. She slowly moves it to the left. I suck in my breath . . . one pound, a pound and three quarters, two pounds, two and a half . . . "You've lost three!" she says, and I let out a whoop. Given the cost of a week at camp, each pound costs, more or less, $200, so weight gain would have been a financial loss.

When I get back to the other room, my friends gather, curious. Although competition is frowned upon ("You're only competing with yourself!" we're told), whenever anyone emerges from the weigh-in room she is greeted with a chorus of, *How'd you do?* and *How much did you lose?* If the verdict is good, we're thrilled to admit it. If it's bad, no one even needs to ask—tears stream down our faces.

A few minutes later Steph comes out. She is smiling; she's lost two pounds. "Last week, I must have been bloated from my period," she says. We give each other high fives. We've both just aced our exams.

After all the campers have been weighed and measured, the counselors get on the scale, a mandatory camp rule. Except for the occasional nutrition or psych major who's here simply for academic purposes, most of the counselors also want to slim down. Many are former campers, and they're all required to follow the program. On weigh-in day the female counselors (ages seventeen plus) strip down to skimpy bathing suits or leotards, squeezing the fat rolls on their stomachs and thighs. They carry their egglet and bagelet in plastic cups, saving them until after weigh-in. They go to the bathroom at least three times, trying desperately to flush all extraneous fluids from their system. The guys joke among themselves, laughing guiltily about the amount of food they consumed on their nights off. They, too, worry about their weight loss, although they know it's nearly impossible for them to gain. Everyone knows men lose weight faster than women, and even when they do go out for "second dinners" (whole pizza pies, meatball subs, hot fudge sundaes), they're still eating half of what they normally would at home.

And so it goes. Some counselors step off the scale happy; others are afraid of Tony Sparber. Though he doesn't care what a counselor does on his or her own time, anyone who brings "non-program" food on campus, or gives extra food to a camper, or gains weight, will be kicked out, no questions asked. Sparber is militant about that, and so all bingeing takes place secretly, on days off or late at night when the kids are asleep. Some adventurous counselors hide nachos or Doritos in the bottom of their duffel bags; others lock chocolate in their closet. But no one fools anyone: The campers, like police dogs trained to sniff out marijuana, can smell food from a mile away. And Sparber himself has been known to rummage through suspicious counselors' belongings in search of candy bars, cookies, or cakes. He rarely comes out empty-handed.

» «

Most of us know that, at its core, losing weight is a physiological process. You ingest fewer calories, you lose pounds. Period. If psychology—and, to a certain extent, biology—didn't enter into the picture, of course, we'd all be thin. The beauty of the fat camp is that it is an environment that eliminates psychology and free will and focuses mostly on the physiological piece: an artificial universe where every meal is preprepared, regulated, and monitored. It is almost—but not completely—impossible to deviate from the rules. If you stick to the program, you will lose weight.

That, at least, is the hope of campers and their parents: that fat camp will be a one-time fix, and that the camper will lose enough weight in one pop to be motivated to stay thin forever; that it will provide a crash course in nutrition—or, at least, a two-month hiatus from weight *gain*, giving everyone involved a respite from the anxiety and battles.

But what fat camp doesn't address are the emotional and familial components that contribute to obesity—at least, not in any real way. Camps provide technical information on weight loss, but they don't adequately address the emotional issues. For most kids—for most *people*—technical information isn't enough.

When you step on the grounds of a fat farm, the outside world ceases to exist. Everything shifts out of balance, size becomes relative, and objects in the mirror are usually larger than they appear. You don't realize it, though. Stephanie calls it "fat goggles"—an apt description for the unique optical illusion created at fat camp. When you're surrounded by people who weigh 200, 250 pounds, everything seems small in comparison. Those who weigh 180 are at the lighter end of the spectrum; a 160-pounder is downright slender.

A fat farm is also a place where the extra flab on your body no longer distinguishes you from the crowd. Call out "Hey, Fatso!" and fifty people are going to turn around. There's something comforting about this, a camaraderie I imagine war veterans understand.

When I was fifteen my grandfather died, leaving me a sizable inheritance. I decided to spend some of the extra cash on a weight-loss camp, or food rehab, as I liked to think of it.

An acquaintance of mine lost twenty-five pounds at Camp Colang and looked great. Never mind that three months later she'd gained it all back, plus ten. I knew that the only place I'd ever get thin was somewhere without an easily accessible bulk-food section, where there were other people trapped in the same miserable, oversized barge. It seemed perfect, a haven for "overweight men and women to make good friends and build self-esteem in the heart of the pines and the Poconos," as the brochures used to say. Sure, it was expensive—about $3,500 for nine weeks, money I could have put toward college—but I thought it was worth it, and I happily forked over the cash.

I never discussed my plans with friends. It seemed embarrassing, too easy an out, and I didn't want to admit that I needed this . . . *fat farm* to help me lose weight. I figured I'd tell them I'd had mono all summer and had gotten skinny as a result. I couldn't wait to go to camp, couldn't wait to go back home and lead a different (read: happier, better, party- and boy-filled) life. How would it not be? I'd be thin.

And being thin was what it was all about. But not too thin. The night before I left for Colang, my sister and I were standing in the kitchen. My mother turned to her and said, "You're too thin, you've got to gain weight!" Then she swiveled my way and said, "You've got to lose weight, you have a double chin!" I was furious and a huge fight ensued, with my sister shrieking, "She's going to a *fat farm?*" The next day I flew alone to Scranton, Pennsylvania, and cried the whole way there. (A journal entry from that flight: "Here I am, en route to Anorexicville . . .")

As soon as I arrived at camp I was greeted by a bunch of hefty people in red T-shirts tossing around a Frisbee. I vividly remember thinking: *What did I get myself into?*

Back in 1984, I was five foot two and 136 pounds. Hardly a heifer. But according to those now-defunct life insurance charts (and my parents) I should have been twenty-six pounds lighter. I believed them, just as I believed my life would turn around once the excess poundage disappeared. Just as I believed that fat camp would cure all my problems. Fat people, after all, were weak, without willpower or self-control. And who wanted to be thought of that way? Of course, the real problem wasn't the weight. The weight was a symptom of unhappiness, sadness, loneliness. But it became a problem because this culture accepts mental illness a lot better than it does fat.

So I went to Camp Colang—colon with a g, as I liked to say— high in the Pocono Mountains. It was lush, sprawling, secluded, the perfect setting for a group of social outcasts to congregate. And we *were* outcasts: ten-year-old kids who weighed over one hundred pounds, adults who weighed-in at 260, and one girl, Maria Scarpelli, who tipped the scales at 350. I was clearly one of the smaller people, which turned me into a worse sort of pariah, too big for the real world, too small for the fat farm. (While I was not the typical fat-farm camper, kids like me who were a few pounds overweight were almost more worrisome than the obese kids because we really had no business being at camp. We were chasing an impossible beauty ideal, and most of us would spend our lives grappling with eating disorders and weight obsession—fueled, I would argue, by the camps.) Before sending in my application I'd half-wondered if there was a weight requirement, if you had to be at least forty pounds overweight before the directors would let you in. But I do not know of any fat-checker who refused you admittance if you were too small. There was no such thing as too small—people would always be fat, and they would always do, and pay, anything to lose weight.

» «

On the first day of camp my counselor, Suzanne, led me to the Bison Bunk, home for the next nine weeks. I laughed when I saw the sign, and wondered why a weight-loss camp had named a cabin for buffalo when its campers were self-conscious enough as it was. Today I wonder if this was supposed to be empowering, like homosexuals calling themselves queer. Were we supposed to be Taking Back Fat? This seems unlikely, since one of the things Suzanne told the twenty-five campers in my bunk was that though we were obviously all heavy, we were not supposed to acknowledge this fact. "We get enough of that out there," she'd said, nodding past the pine trees and soccer field to the road. "This place is about acceptance."

At the time, I was impressed. *Finally,* a community where who we were, not what we looked like, counted. Today the irony of Suzanne's speech strikes me. We weren't at camp to learn to be happy with our bodies; we had just shelled out thousands of dollars to *change* them. We were trying to eradicate the one thing we all had in common. We hated ourselves; our fat, we believed, had caused all of our misery and grief. Indeed, not once in the nine weeks I was at camp would anyone say that it was okay to be overweight. Why would they?

6

Weight-loss camps are, above all else, huge moneymaking machines, and without weaklings like us, how would they survive?

While I unpacked, Suzanne hovered over me, surreptitiously glancing into my suitcase as I tossed clothes onto my bed. Later I learned that counselors had been forewarned as to which kids could be trusted and which couldn't, who was a food felon and who wasn't. Food smuggling did happen: A ten-year-old-boy had stuffed a bag of Hershey's Kisses into the mouth of his tuba. The chocolate was later confiscated (read: inhaled) by his counselors, but the boy was lauded throughout camp for his ingenuity.

I never understood this behavior. We were there to lose weight. Why deliberately sabotage it? But then I realized that I was an anomaly. Most of the campers weren't there of their own free will. Most had been sent by parents who couldn't bear to look at their fat children, by parents whose kids reminded them of their own inadequacies. Most of the campers, I soon learned, didn't give a hoot about losing weight; that is, they wanted desperately to be skinny, but not enough to stop eating the good stuff. They hoped that by simply stepping on camp grounds their fat cells would miraculously disappear.

Maybe if the campers had learned self-acceptance, there wouldn't have been so many repeat customers. The rate of return was high. We may have lost weight during the summer, but our behaviors didn't change when we went back to our pre-fat-farm existence. How could they? Who does aerobics and calisthenics six mornings a week and swims, runs, and hikes six afternoons? Who munches celery sticks instead of Kit Kats? And perhaps more importantly, how many people's families are really willing to change the entire household to accommodate the child in need? I swore I wouldn't be like that. For me, camp would be a one-shot deal: Take one summer, lose thirty pounds, and never come back. Ha! It's easy to lose weight in a controlled environment. It's a different story when you're on your own.

Besides, Colang didn't try to address the real reasons we were fat. Oh, we had rap sessions twice a week, but no one took them seriously. We could have used a camp therapist, but she would have gone mad. So much pain and unhappiness. At midnight gab sessions my bunk mates and I shared the unhappy stories behind our overeating—family traumas, custody battles, sexual abuse. Camp may have covered the wounds with a Band-Aid, but it never let them breathe and heal. Naturally, those of us who used food as a substitute for love, affection, and attention would continue to do so in the real world. Camp may have enabled us to lose weight, but it didn't improve our self-esteem or help us deal with our developing bodies and powerful emotions. Camp attempted the impossible by trying to change a lifetime of learned habits in two months.

So what did we focus on? Food. Being deprived takes its toll. My friends and I spent hours—literally, hours—mapping out what we were going to eat once we got back to the real world. At dinner we'd toy with our broiled fish or calf's liver and tantalize each other with talk of pizza and hot dogs and French fries smothered in ketchup. At night, we wanted to know what was for breakfast; in the morning, the first thing we wondered about was lunch. Like sex-deprived soldiers who pinned up posters of Betty Grable during World War II, we taped up photos of cakes and cookies on the bunk wall, right next to pictures of models from the *Sports Illustrated* swimsuit issue. We envied their bodies almost as much as we lusted for junk food.

Sometimes, we acted on our longings. Once, after I gained half a pound for no apparent reason, my counselor Elaine, a three-year camp veteran who had lost and relost sixty pounds, decided to take matters into her own hands. "Your system needs to be shaken up," she explained. "Your body's getting used to the diet. You need sugar to give it a jolt."

I'd never heard that kind of logic before, but it sounded good to me. At eleven o'clock that night I slipped on a hooded back sweat suit and snuck into the parking lot where Elaine kept her Chevy Nova. We sped off to the Grand Union, terrified and elated.

Elaine was, after all, risking her job. She could get fired for taking a camper off grounds and, more importantly, feeding her. I could have been kicked out of camp with no refund. Or worse, Tony Sparber might have called my folks—protocol when kids were caught in the act.

Elaine and I pulled up to the supermarket. I waited in the produce section, huddled against a wall, while she scoped the store for other camp people. It had been weeks since I'd been in the real world; I felt like a paroled felon about to commit grand larceny. I was convinced *Fat Farm Defector* was scrawled all over me and that the cashier knew I was engaged in highly illegal activities. Happily, no alarms sounded and Elaine and I calmly filled our cart with Mallomars and chocolate-chip cookie dough and Three Musketeers and Reese's Pieces and the requisite six-pack of Diet Coke. Elaine paid the bill while my system geared up for the big jolt. We didn't even wait to get into the car before tearing open the packages. Within an hour I was left with a pile of wrappers and a bout of diarrhea.

But it worked. The following week I stepped on the scale: I'd lost two pounds.

Not everyone snuck away from camp like I did. Other kids raided the dining hall in the middle of the night, stealing jars of peanut butter, loaves of bread, and, the all time coup, Weight Watchers ice cream. They'd hide the food in the rafters and throw a party. And what went on at a fat-camp party? Excessive chowing, discussions about excessive chowing, or a hearty combination of the two.

There was also a black market of food at Colang, an underground ring of food smugglers. Money-hungry counselors knew that campers would pay $5 for a Snickers bar, $4 for a hoagie, $2.75 for a bag of chips (inflation has since elevated the price). They knew the campers were desperate, that we lived for the day when we could go out and buy our own piles of goodies. It was all we thought about, and I would argue that those of us who didn't have eating disorders when we arrived at camp, certainly had developed them by the time we left. The former director of Camp California, a Weight Watchers Camp in Los Olivos, California, where I briefly worked in the early 1990s, told me, "I eat what I want during the year and end up gaining weight because I know I'm going to be at camp all summer."

Even Tony Sparber himself, the Man about Camp, usually came back chubbier.

At night everyone gathered in the "Castle," a building that divided the girls' section of camp (Upper Camp) from the boys' (Lower Camp). Here you could purchase, at additional fees, magazines, icies (an ice cube filled with low-cal soda), and sugarless gum. Gum was a fat-farm staple. Since it wasn't really considered a food, we were allowed to have it. We chewed it by the pack, popping piece after piece into our mouths before the last one had lost its flavor. We always needed something to suck on, and we'd sneak cigarettes when we weren't chewing or eating or drinking caseloads of Crystal Light.

For me, camp was a bastion of mixed messages. On the one hand, I was healthier—physically, anyway—than I'd been in years. But psychologically I was getting sicker and sicker. Not only did I start actively smoking after my first summer there, I also chewed wads of sugared gum, which my counselors bought for me. Once I plowed through eighteen packs of Bubble Yum in less than three hours, shoving piece after piece into my mouth. Two years later I had a root canal. (Today most camps ban sugared gum, though of course kids manage to get it).

And competition was fierce. If campers—and counselors, most of whom were just a year or two older than the oldest campers—weren't competing to see who could consume the most food and still lose weight, then we were competing socially. Unfortunately, the most popular kids were the thinner ones. My 350-pound friend Maria, for example, was often teased because she snored, because she walked so slowly, because she was *just so goddamned fat.* Another girl had fallen through her bed, breaking the frame and board. Soon the story made its way around camp. The hypocrisy infuriated me, that people were ridiculed about their weight at a fat farm, but it was merely a microcosm of the real world, where there's no escaping it. The pressure to look good and be the prettiest, the thinnest, the most popular seems to be everywhere, even in places where you'd think it wouldn't.

We competed for weight loss, too. It was ludicrous—someone who weighs 180 pounds is bound to lose more weight than someone forty pounds lighter—but we'd compare ourselves nonetheless. When one of us had a bad weight loss we'd pat her on the back: "You lost a pound and a half—be psyched!" all the while feeling smug because, damn it, we'd lost a pound and *three-quarters*.

And just as girls have done since the biblical days of Leah and Rachel, we battled for boys—boys we would never have even sniffed at elsewhere. Camp was coed, with a sixty-forty female to male split. The lack of testosterone meant the boys had us girls eating out of the palms of their hands—not a particularly difficult feat for a group of hungry kids. At socials, the skinnier girls would always get asked to dance, while the heavier ones sat on the benches and watched. I had more boys interested in me that summer than I ever had before—or since, actually. It was the first time in my life that guys seemed attracted to me and told me how cute I was, how well built. The irony didn't escape me—and God knows I would have resented myself had the tables been turned—but I sucked it all up like a sugar swizzle.

Despite this rivalry, we campers did share a bond, a camaraderie that those who haven't been overweight can never really understand. Though I may not have known what it was like to be obese, I, like everyone else there, knew what it was like to be teased—you don't get called Flabby Abby for nothing—and to feel inadequate because my body was less than perfect. There was a support network at camp. When some little hobbit-like guy dumped one of us, we could always find a friendly shoulder to cry on. And when one of us tired in aerobics, someone was always there to spur us on. To this day, some of my closest friends are from camp.

As it happened, Colang was one of three specialized camps in the area: one for mentally challenged kids, one for juvenile delinquents, and then us, the fatties. My friend Sean used to joke, "Watch your money, your toys, and your food."

» «

Fat camps have changed somewhat since I was a kid—mostly financially (they cost about $7,000 a summer, compared to $3,500 back in the 1980s), though also in terms of food. Whereas in the past we talked about going on a diet, or sticking to a diet, or cheating from our diet, the conversation these days is on healthy eating and portion control. It doesn't matter, of course—kids still feel deprived, and they still obsess about food, and they still plot their post-camp meals with gusto. So what does this mean for you, the parent of a child who's just returned from camp? That there's a good chance your child will gain his weight back at a fairly rapid clip, and there's not much you can do about it. It's not your fault; your child is simply set up for failure from the minute he walks into camp.

In the weight-loss-camp world—which is, like most subcultures, fairly insular—Tony Sparber is both feared and revered. It's understandable. He can be gruff and combative, and he's not afraid to voice his opinions. When I first met him he seemed to have a rage gurgling about one centimeter beneath the surface. His crudeness is sort of his trademark, and the people around him know that you either play by his rules or you don't play at all.

Tony Sparber is six foot four and now, at forty-seven, slightly beefy, with an angular jaw, long incisors, and a receding dark hairline flecked with gray. He reigns over his camp with the hubris of Donald Trump. He often refers to his domain as Sparberland; he is Lord of the Farm, the Grand Poobah of Fat World. He guarantees that campers will leave "in the best physical and mental shape of their lives." Thousands of kids—including, it was rumored, Kim Fields, the girl who played Tootie on *The Facts of Life,* and Gladys Knight's son, Shanga—have spent summers with him, lifting weights, stepping on scales, and obsessing about food. In certain circles, he is legendary.

Despite his shortcomings, in a strange way I feel like he's family—albeit more like the long-lost relative you're happy to see, say, once every seven years. For better or for worse, Tony Sparber is responsible for some of the most important experiences of my life.

(I'm not sure that these events were necessarily good, in the grand scheme of things, but that is getting ahead of the story.)

As is the case at most summer camps, Tony's life was dissected ad nauseam. He could be mean, and instilled a terrible fear in his campers and counselors. He talked—and still does—like a street kid, his language pickled with *yo*s and *man*s and *whassup*s long before they became part of the vernacular. He wasn't one, though—he grew up in a three-bedroom apartment on Washington Square Park in Manhattan, and went to the ultra-liberal Little Red School House and Elizabeth Irwin High School, where he felt horribly misplaced. He was surrounded by commies and hippies, but he was a jock. "I had a miserable childhood," he admits. "I couldn't wait to move to the suburbs. I always wanted structure."

Since he couldn't relate to the EI radicals, he'd head to the Sixth Avenue basketball courts to shoot hoops with the homeboys. He penetrated their world as much as possible, but there were, quite naturally, barriers that prevented a white Jewish kid from fully bonding with the dudes from the 'hood. He was lonely and sad, and to combat his insecurities he developed a persona of intolerance.

"I was a little bit overweight and I used to tell my parents I was going out to a party, but instead I'd just walk the streets of New York," he says. "It was embarrassing."

His father, Mike, ran Weight Watchers camps around the country. Tony literally grew up at summer camp—he went to his first one at age four—and throughout the years held a variety of positions at Colang, including head of the kitchen at seventeen, and head counselor at twenty-one.

At twenty-seven, Tony took over Colang, one of twelve Weight Watchers camps ran by the Sparbers. Although we did follow the Weight Watchers program, the camps were not run by them. Sparber had to pay Weight Watchers a 10 percent licensing fee for the name. Colang was the only traditional camp of the lot. The others were on college campuses. (The Colang property has had many incarnations—my mother went there in the 1950s when it was a girls' camp; now it's a resort for Hasidic kids.) His father sold the business three years later, and Tony was given a five-year contract with the new owners.

Five years later, he says he received a letter saying that his services were no longer needed. "It was 1992. I'd gotten married in '86 and my wife was pregnant and here I am with no job," he says. "I was a little bitter. I was supposed to be like most Jewish men's sons and take over the family business, but when I got to that point the family business wasn't there anymore. It got sold right out from under me."

He panicked. His marriage suffered. (He met his wife, Dale, when she was a Colang counselor; she had always envisioned herself as "Queen of the Weight Watchers camp," he says. "She was really thrown when this happened.")

Still, whatever doesn't kill you makes you stronger, and that he is. After he left Colang, which closed as a weight-loss camp two years later, Sparber found a property in Connecticut and brought on two longtime Colang campers-turned-counselors, Tricia Winfield and Tammy Weinstein, to help recruit kids. About eighty children signed on and Tony Sparber's New Image opened its doors. In 1995, he took over facilities in Florida and California. By 1997, he realized he no longer needed the Connecticut camp, and he found the spot in Pennsylvania. This past summer, over 1,000 kids attended his three New Image camps.

» «

Tony Sparber's Camp Pocono Trails sits on a magnificent parcel of land in Readers, Pennsylvania, about an hour from where Colang used to be. I'd always thought Colang was beautiful—100 acres, in the backyard of the Delaware River, where we'd inner tube, sneak cigarettes, or party with people we met rafting—but this was magnificent. Sparber leases it for the summer; he says he doesn't want the headache of owning a place. At 350 acres, the camp has climbing walls, two huge swimming pools, a lake, and spacious cabins with single beds—no embarrassing bunk beds—complete with maid service.

I had not seen this man since 1990, my last year at Colang, and frankly, I was nervous. There's always an element of trepidation when you see anyone from the fat farm era, even—or especially—twenty years later. You want people to think you're different, that you defied the odds and were actually a success (read: thin). And I admit it, I wanted his approval. He was a father figure to so many kids, many of whom ached for any kind of authority figure.

No one, perhaps, more than Stephanie Winston.

I met Stephanie my first year at Colang. She was legendary, with her shoulder-length platinum blonde hair, tattoos on her ankles and upper back, and enormous breasts (38 DD!). She was eighteen—two years older than me—and lived with the older girls in the so-called Collegiate House, a big rust-colored dormitory in the middle of camp. Collegiates had special privileges—they always ate first, for example, and got to take field trips to the Middletown Mall, while everyone else had to stay at camp. Her great-grand uncle was Harry Winston, the diamond peddler, and she grew up a spoiled New York brat on Park Avenue. At camp, she brought her own electric fan and boom box; she drove a Trans Am with a GTYRWNGS license plate (an ode to Aerosmith, not Colonel Sanders). I used to watch her carry her guitar down to the river with some hot counselor, looking like she'd jumped right out of *Fast Times at Ridgemont High*, and I never understood what the hell she was doing at camp. She seemed too cool for it.

Steph and I didn't become friends until my second year, when I lived in Collegiate House. We were both Deadheads, both smoked Marlboro Lights, both were too small for the fat farm but too big for the real world. What I hadn't known was that Stephanie had spent ages thirteen to fifteen shuttling from one hospital to another. Her mother had been dying from a brain tumor (she died when Steph was fifteen) and her father relied on alcohol to get through the pain, and then on rehab centers to get through the reliance. Little Miss Cool was desperately unhappy; she had no parental supervision and lost herself in sex, drugs, rock 'n' roll, and Chipwiches. (My second year of camp, six out of the ten girls in my bunks had deceased mothers.) Apparently, the kids at school teased her mercilessly; she looked to camp for self-esteem. She needed an authority figure and Tony Sparber fit the bill. But she was always getting into trouble for things, like smoking cigarettes or sunbathing down at the river when she was supposed to be playing volleyball.

My first year, Stephanie had been promoted from camper to counselor. She didn't especially want the responsibility, but she was dating a counselor, and since camper/counselor relationships were verboten, she figured it made sense to rise to his level. (A camp maxim: Male counselors rule the roost. Sparber has joked that in his next life, "I want to come back as a guy counselor in Lower Camp.")

One night near the end of Color War, a four-day-long all-camp competition that Sparber oversees with McNamarian precision, Stephanie took a camper friend, Heather, out to a bar where the counselors hung out at night. Sparber barged in the door, took one look at Heather and Stephanie, and bellowed, "You and you, come with me!"

He sent Steph home early, with just four days left of camp, and the event was so traumatic she spent the next twenty years dreaming about Tony Sparber looming over her at the bar, foaming at the mouth like a rabid dog. He likes this version of himself. "Fear is what differentiates this camp from others," he says. "The kids are afraid of me."

He took her back the next year, of course—why turn down $3,500?—and I think he genuinely liked Stephanie. He saw something of himself in her. They were both from the city, both attracted to people who were not of their social class, and both very, very sad.

He even let her work for him again. At the time there were Weight Watchers camps all over the country, on college campuses in Massachusetts, California, Florida, and Long Island. (This was a big thing. Camp Camelot and Camp La Jolla also operated weight-loss camps on college campuses.) Steph and I were counselors together on the Hampshire College campus in Northampton, Massachusetts, on the North Adams State College campus, and back at Colang in 1990.

When I told Stephanie that I was going to visit Tony's new camp, she jumped at the chance to see him.

"I want to exorcise him from my psyche!" she said earnestly.

Interestingly, despite her Sparber phobia, she only saw camp as a positive. It was "where I discovered my real self because I could never be my real self in the real world," she said. "I never could express myself in ways where I wouldn't be made fun of, and I never felt able to just . . . shine. I remember this guy in high school getting mad at me and calling me a 'fat f**k.'"

"I find that so hard to believe," I said. "You were, like, Queen of the Farm."

"Which gave me great self-esteem," she said. "But everybody in my school was thin and rich and I was the outcast." (Well, size-wise, anyway.)

To this day, she is haunted by Chipwiches, by memories of "leaving school at the end of the day, going to the deli around the corner, getting a Chipwich and knowing that that's all I wanted. That was my vice. In eleventh grade I got fat on Chipwiches. Chipwiches possess me. Along with Sparber."

I laughed. I didn't feel that way about him; he amused me, actually. Every Sunday, weigh-in day, he serenaded the entire camp with his rendition of "Zipadee-Doo-Dah." ("My, oh my, well it's weigh-in day. Plenty of poundage, going away. . . .") And he was good to me. In 1986, my second and fattest year (147 pounds!), I could only afford seven weeks at Colang. Once again I'd used my own money, and I simply didn't have enough. I didn't want to go home, though, and so Sparber arranged for me to stay on as babysitter to the three-year-old son of the camp nurse. It was a lovely gesture, which I still appreciate.

Still, when I called him and told him I wanted to come see him, I was apprehensive. I didn't know what he would say, if he would even remember me or if he would hate me for having published an article in the now-defunct *Mademoiselle* about my experiences at Camp Colang. But he was nice and asked me to get back in touch in a few weeks, once camp started.

» «

"Holy cow!" Stephanie exclaims when we drive up to the gate of Pocono Trails. We spot Sparber in the distance, and we both giggle nervously, like we are eighteen years old and fat.

After hugging us hello, Tony motions for us to sit down in his office. We laugh about how weird it is to see each other after so many years (it's June 2003). At first, he doesn't even recognize Stephanie, so vast is her transformation from insecure young teen to moderately together adult. She looks completely different: Her hair is its natural brown, cropped short like Demi Moore's in *Ghost,* and she wears glasses. She had a breast reduction and weighs about 110 pounds. Me, he knew. I'm smaller, but I still wear glasses and not a lot of makeup and look pretty much the same. "You guys have been successful," he says. "You've done well." We beam.

He offers us Diet Coke and bottled water, and launches into the saga of how his camp came to be. It's strange to be sitting with him after all these years, like when you finally become friends with a college professor and you realize that the Wizard is really just some dude.

Like Colang, Sparber's camps are comprised mostly of white Jewish kids from New Jersey, Pennsylvania, and Florida. About 650 spend the summer in Pennsylvania; the number rises to 1,000 with his two other camps in Florida and California. Seven and a half weeks costs $7,000—about the same as any good regular camp, he says. About ten to fifteen kids are on scholarship.

"Colang was a zoo," he admits, and we each chuckle at our own memories. "Once a guy came in off the river, and walked right onto camp grounds. We didn't know him from Adam, but he was thin, and so we hired him. Crazy."

He blames much of the chaos on himself. He was too young—twenty-five, twenty-six—to be running a camp and disciplining an older staff.

And the kids were different back then. Kids today are much mellower. "They're all about the American flag, they have more respect, and they're more responsible. The selfishness is gone. They're a lot more compassionate." This could be the result of 9/11, he hypothesizes, or it could be because more of them take Prozac, Lithium, Ritalin, or Adderal. Not that these kids are any more screwed up than most kids in the country—they just wear their troubles on their bodies.

"Directors at traditional camps would tell you that in the traditional population there is an increase in meds and in kids who come from dysfunctional families," says Lucy J. Norvell, director of Public Information for the American Camping Association of New England.

The number of male campers at fat camps has also increased, as has the percentage of younger kids, ages seven, eight, and nine. And kids all over the country are bigger. "We went to a water park on Thursday and it was really weird, because in the past when you went to the water park you would be able to pick out our kids, you knew exactly who they were," Sparber says. "Now you can't tell who are our kids and who aren't."

The other thing is that about 95 percent of the kids want to come. In the past, their parents would force them to go to camp, but now it's their choice.

As always, many of the children are products of divorce, and many have fat parents who send mixed messages ("Eat! Be thin! Eat!"). On visiting day, some parents take the kids off grounds and they pig out as a unit. Although the camp offers a nutrition lecture for families, only about half of them actually attend.

"The people who are successful are the parents who go the extra mile and are observant and watching their kids," Sparber says. "Unfortunately, there are a lot of kids who don't have both parents at home, and a lot of these kids have no limits at all. The exposure these kids have—what TV shows they're allowed to watch, what they're allowed to look at, the MTV and the reality shows. One's worse than the next. There's basically no control at home over what they can watch or what they can do. Up here it's different. We do really believe in responsibility. They've got to make their beds, they've got to clean up, they've got to go to activities. They are definitely held to a higher standard here than they are at home, and that I think is a big thing."

He also extols the social value of camp. "A lot of kids here have no social lives to speak of at home, and here they're completely accepted. One of the things we don't tolerate is any type of bullying or people being mean to other people. We sent a couple of kids home for that. We'll call the parents and tell them, 'Listen, if your child's behavior doesn't change and if it happens again we'll send them out.'" I think even more important than weight loss is the emotional growth that the kids get from a place like this.

"To me it's very gratifying," Sparber continues. "I have tremendous compassion for these kids. It's a great position and I love helping them, but it's very intense. At camp you see people for who they are. You see them without their makeup on. You see them in the morning, at night. There's no facade. I think camp is one of the last areas that's pure. The biggest challenge is trying to keep that pure environment. Keeping the outside influences outside of the camp is an ongoing battle, especially with a camp this size. I'm talking about parents smuggling in cell phones when I tell them not to or sending their kids things they aren't supposed to. There are many enablers out there. Parents don't know how to say no to their kids. They don't know how to set any limits or boundaries."

Once the summer ends he offers after-care programs with personal training and nutritional counseling on Long Island and in New Jersey. Do people come? "It starts out strong and then as time goes on it fades," he says. "We have a couple of nutritionists on retainer during the year; they call up the kids and do on-the-phone counseling. The only problem with that is that when we call them and leave messages and some call back and some don't. The truth is—and I tell everybody this—if you don't live in New Jersey or Long Island where we are, you must find something locally. I cannot give them the magic answer. There has to be something hands-on and you have to make an effort. There are plenty of trainers, plenty of nutritionists, there are Weight Watcher classrooms in all the areas. Get down there and do something instead of saying 'I can't find something, I'm too busy.' Parents who make the effort to find something—those kids are much more successful. And the kids who train with us for the most part are very successful long term."

Tony hands Stephanie and me a baseball cap with the words *Pocono Trails* emblazoned on the bill—we're psyched!—and the three of us tour the camp. It really is Sparberland. The kids call out and run up to him. He waves back—"You're lookin' good, keep it up!" He knows every kid by name, in addition to things you wouldn't expect him to know, like the fact that Jane Bauer, a thirteen-year-old with short blonde hair, a puffy face, and small eyes, had lied to me about her weight.

I'd run into her by a field where the entire camp was engaged in an intense game of Capture the Flag, a Sparber favorite. But Jane wasn't playing; she'd hurt her knee and couldn't run. This was her third year at camp; so far she'd lost twenty-nine and a half pounds in six weeks, but she freely admitted that she gained it back after.

I asked how much she weighed. "Two sixty-five," she replied—which Tony overheard.

"She's 300," he told me later. "She was embarrassed. But don't put that in the story." (I told him I wouldn't use her real name, and I haven't.)

Later, Stephanie, Tony, and I eat lunch—turkey sandwiches on a real bun, coleslaw, a gorgeous, fresh salad bar, and an ice cream popsicle—and talk more about how camp has changed in twenty years.

One thing that's different today is that counselors no longer have to weigh in. Sparber doesn't care if they're fat or thin. "Sometimes it's nice having the overweight counselor," he says. "I probably prefer the in-shape guys; their productivity is a little bit higher, to be honest with you, but I don't want to make a generalization because it's not always true. But I will say that some of my overweight counselors really tend to be a little lazy sometimes."

His own schedule is pretty light. From the beginning of April to August 16, when camp ends, he works like a madman; then he, his wife, and son take a vacation. "We get a big suite and just hang out," he says. "I take the month of September off and honestly I don't work very much until April. I coach my son's football and basketball; I'm a very hands-on father. I'm very active in the JCC where I live. I only work hard for seven and a half weeks and then I'm done. I can be a father and I can go home."

He is making a point, and I wonder what he's really trying to say.

"The point I'm trying to make is that eventually these kids are going to find their place in the world. They do. A lot of them grow out of their freakiness."

» «

And a lot don't.

In his forty-odd years on earth, Ted Donnelly has lost and regained nearly 400 pounds, and has spent over twenty years attending or working at weight-loss camps. He is now so heavy he's confined to a wheelchair. Frank Cartwright, forty-three, has spent just about as long doing the same thing. He's thinner than Donnelly—six feet, 260 pounds, tops—but he has never just thrown in the towel and stopped trying to lose weight. It is, he admits, his "mission" in life. He returns to camp year after year, like Charlotte's three offspring in *Charlotte's Web*, who simply can't abandon Wilbur after their mother dies.

Tony Sparber's assistant director, Trish Winfield, thirty-four, was sent to Colang at age fourteen, when she was 230 pounds (she's five foot four). She went for nine years straight, working her way from camper to counselor to group leader and then to assistant director. She lost and regained hundreds of pounds, and a few years ago went to Structure House, the residential weight-loss clinic in Durham, North Carolina. She lived there for twelve months and knocked off one hundred pounds, which she maintained for almost a year. But then she gained it back and more, all the way up to 330 pounds. So she had gastric bypass surgery. "I felt backed against the wall," she says. She looks tired—haggard, really, like she's run a never-ending marathon—with saggy skin and sad eyes. But she's thin. "I had no other choice. I don't think it's the best step, but it has helped me." (She doesn't tell the campers how she lost weight.)

Benjamin Weill is well on his way to becoming just like Donnelly, Cartwright, and Winfield. At seventeen, Ben has been fat—"enormous," as his father, a PR executive, puts it—pretty much his entire life. Camp Shane, in Ferndale, New York, has been his summer home away from home since he was nine.

Camp Shane is situated in just about the worst location a fat camp could be. Oh, it's pretty—green and hilly—but a half a mile down the road there's a gas station, a Taco Bell, McDonald's, Wendy's, Pizza Hut, and Burger King. The campers are well aware of this. Hyper aware. In fact, they have been known to sneak out for a very happy meal.

Like almost everyone I know who has gone to weight-loss camp—or any camp, for that matter—Ben loves it, not so much for the facilities, which are fairly run-down, but for the friends he has made over the years. And it's helped with weight. "I think if I hadn't gone to Shane I'd be significantly heavier than I am and have ever been," he admits. "It did help me keep my weight in check." (But some things are just plain weird, he says, like when the camp hired a fat nutritionist. "I loved that!" says Ben. "Telling us how to eat right and all the things we have to do to lose weight. I thought, 'Really? After all of your experience and time spent testing these methods?'")

Camp is simply a part of him, like his brown eyes, his curly hair, his girth. Unlike many fat people, he doesn't object to the word "fat." That's what he is. Fat.

We are sitting in his family's apartment on the Upper West side, a sunny place filled with Judaic paintings, books, and a terrace with a lovely view of Central Park. Ben sips a Diet Coke and cuddles a cat. His cuticles are scraggly and caked with dried blood; he's nervous about something. Every time he shifts, his end of the couch rises, but he doesn't seem to notice or care.

He's very flamboyant and theatrical, and incredibly outgoing. He loves being the center of attention. In 2002 he starred in an MTV special about weight-loss camps, becoming a celebrity of sorts to fat hipsters everywhere. People recognized him on the street and asked for his autograph, which thrilled him. He has always wanted to act and almost landed a role as the fat kid on the TV show *Ed* except—just his luck—the directors ultimately decided he was too thin. Talk about a bummer.

For a kid who's been obese most of his life, Ben seems fairly well adjusted, especially when you consider the recent changes in his world. Some are good—like the fact that he lost eighty-two pounds during the summer of 2002, going from 386 to 304, which he has kept off for a year and a half, the longest time ever. He has a girl-friend, Kate, with whom he has been in love for four years (they've since broken up). He spent the summer of 2003 in an acting pro-gram at Carnegie Mellon University—the first time since he was nine that he was not at fat camp. Wouldn't you know it—he actually lost six pounds.

"This year is different," he says. "Why? I don't know. I don't want to be this weight." I ask if there's a link between his taking time off to do theater, which he loves, and his maintaining his weight loss. He ponders this. "I'm not obsessing over it and I'm not even think-ing about it. I'm doing stuff that I love to do. Yes, there's a link. Do you know how wonderful it was to go to a place and have people un-derstand what I'm talking about?" (The unstated implication: *And not have it be about my weight?*)

Initially it was strange not being in the familiar Shane cocoon, and he spent the first couple of days at Carnegie Mellon very con-scious of "being big," but never to the point of being uncomfort-able, and "after a couple of days I didn't care," he says. "There are times when I feel self-conscious, like everyone is like, 'Oh look at this fat guy.' Then I think, 'Why would they be wasting their time doing this?'"

Then there are the bad changes, like his parents, who have split up after a volatile and unhappy marriage. His mother is a shrink with her own weight struggles; his father works in public relations and has wrestled with about twenty extra pounds. Although Ben always wished his folks would divorce, he was shocked when they finally told him they were doing it—the day they brought him back from camp, in 2002.

"They said, 'We need to talk to you, we need to tell you something.' Mom is bawling and they tell me what's going to happen. Then we all go to see Dad's house on 54th Street. That's the type of sadistic family I was born into."

Sure, he ate more after his father moved out, possibly because he was angry at him, possibly because "I'm pissed at my mom for trying to replace Dad with me and for nagging and nagging." But there is also this indisputable fact: "I wanted to eat, and I'm sure I used one excuse or the other more times than it was actually fair." He does not drink or smoke. Food is his addiction.

"If you're having a really bad day, just knowing you shouldn't be having this chocolate or whatever makes you feel a little bit better," he says. "Personally, I don't even see the point of cottage cheese."

Ben says he knows what underlying problems cause him to eat. He was first put into therapy for writing suicidal poetry at age nine. He hates shrinks. "The problem with me is I'm either too smart or I just think I am, I haven't decided which one. I never feel like they're going to tell me something I don't know," he says. "I had one therapist whose entire vocabulary consisted of the phrase 'How does that make you feel?' I threatened to kill him. 'How does that make you feel?' I know that I like to eat and I always will. I love to cook. Anything that's involved with food, I love." He has, not surprisingly, entertained the idea of being a chef. But acting is where his heart is; hopefully, his weight won't get in the way.

He is open and thoughtful, but obviously harbors a lot of resentment toward his mother. (Once I called him and she answered. She put him on the phone. I asked how he is, what's going on, and he replied, "Not much!" In the background his mother screamed,

"What do you mean 'not much?' You're applying to school!" He sighed.)

She hounds him relentlessly, he says. Her biggest worry is that Ben will have no opportunities at this size—no one to hire him and no one to love him—which is the fear of all parents of overweight kids. But if you really think about it, that's everyone's fear no matter how much they weigh.

Other than poor endurance and some joint problems, he has no health problems, he says. Not quite true, says his mom.

Ben was born with a clubfoot. He had surgery when he was five, was in a cast for eight weeks, and started gaining weight. His mom isn't sure if the weight gain was the result of the foot problem, the inactivity, or his depression, which debuted around the same time. After his parents found suicidal poetry he had written he was placed on antidepressants and weight-loss pills: Meridia, Wellbutrin, Topamax, Centromin. He has seen every nutritionist and obesity specialist in Manhattan. Nothing but Camp Shane worked, though that was temporary.

"You can't teach self-control," he says. "I think you can train it, though. You just learn to support yourself, to say no and choose something else. But it has to be your decision. Let the kid decide. He's got to do it. No one can make the choice. Unless you're going to cement his mouth closed, he's going to find a way to eat behind your back. Parents can help push kids in the right direction. They can say, 'Are you sure you want to have another portion?' or 'Are you sure you want to do this or do that?' Or they can say, 'Don't do that, you're going to ruin your life!' Stay away from the latter one."

Fair enough. But I have one more question for him: "Who's responsible for your weight problem?"

For once Ben doesn't have a quip ready to fly off his tongue. "I never thought about that," he says finally. "I don't think any one person. I was born into a family that loves food."

» «

26

The first weight-loss camp in the world for kids was Camp Na-panoch, founded in 1963, in Napanoch, New York. That was di-rected by a woman named Selma Ettenberg, and went out of business three years later. Around the same time Ettenberg hap-pened on a beautiful patch of land in the Catskill Mountains. She took one look and cried out, "What a shayne place!" ("Shayne" is Yiddish for pretty.) She bought it, morphed it into Shane, and in 1968 an industry was born.

Weight-loss camps peaked in 1988, with eighty-four camps. To-day, of the 2,300 camps accredited with the American Camping As-sociation, only six specialize in weight loss, though there are many that are not ACA-accredited. (No one seems to be able to say why there were so many in 1988. Some people in the field speculate that many camps listed themselves as weight-loss even though they weren't.)

Fat camps have slowly woven their way into the international market. In the early 1990s, China opened its first camp for fat ur-ban children, called the Beijing Tian Yu Weight-Loss Camp. Eng-land followed in 1999 with the Carnegie International Weight Loss camp at Leeds Metropolitan University. But a handful of camps that operated in Canada closed up shop in the 1980s, after a grow-ing awareness of anorexia nervosa made them seem "politically in-correct," a spokeswoman for the Canadian Camping Association said.

Statistics on weight-loss camps are hard to come by. The num-bers are difficult to gauge since many people don't respond honestly to surveys. Camp directors most likely jack up the success rates; un-fortunately, there's no real scientific data to prove it one way or the other. In a 1987 follow-up survey, Camp Camelot found that 75 per-cent of graduates who answered a progress report had maintained their weight loss a year later. The figure for the same period was 82 percent among La Jolla graduates. While I had no access to their numbers, my unscientific, anecdotal evidence makes me suspicious.

If you live in New York, New Jersey, or Connecticut, and your child is overweight, chances are you've heard of Camp Shane. Shane has gotten more publicity than most of the other weight-loss camps. The reasons for this are somewhat basic. For one thing, it's only an hour and forty-five minutes from Manhattan, media central. The camp also has a very impressive Web site and video. (Although in person, the place itself feels like it's thirty-five years old. It's over-crowded and a little run-down, with peeling paint on the bunks and structures that look like they're about ready to collapse. The camp owns seven motorboats, but there's no waterfront. Instead, the kids are shuttled to a lake about twenty minutes away.)

Ten years ago, Selma Ettenberg's son, David, took over Camp Shane. (Some people say it was a hostile takeover; Ettenberg himself won't talk about it, and as it happens, he now faces fourteen months in jail for tax fraud.) David Ettenberg is thin, springy, and quite genial, with the demeanor of a car salesman: likable, but you're not quite sure he isn't selling you a lemon. His words tumble out in a torrent. The father of a girl and a boy, both of whom spend their summers at regular camp, he and his wife, Ziporah, run Shane full time from their home in Westchester county, New York. Unlike Tony Sparber, he doesn't instill fear in his campers. In fact, he seems to be almost an afterthought to them. He doesn't seem to know the kids' names; he looks a little bewildered when they call out to him.

Ettenberg, fifty-seven, welcomes media. His camp has been featured on *Dr. Phil, 20/20,* Sally Jesse, and in a host of print magazines. He's also a savvy marketer. He has used the same print ad—a black-and-white photo of a young boy holding his shorts, which are four sizes too large, in front of him—for almost thirty years. "At one point we thought about changing it, but he's an icon," Ettenberg says.

But the real boon came in 2001, when MTV shot its *Real Life: I'm Going to Fat Camp!* at Shane, which garnered such press that Etten-berg says he had to turn kids away. Camp Shane always sells out; there are three sessions lasting three, six, and nine weeks. There's room for about 500 kids and 200 staff. About twenty-five to fifty kids are on financial aid, David says, though none of the parents I spoke to knew about this option.

Calories hover around 1,500, although the kids naturally complain that it's not enough. That makes sense, when you consider what they're used to eating on a normal day at home. The average weight loss per summer is thirty-five pounds. The average weight gain during the school year is about forty.

Ettenberg is philosophical about the high rate of return. The way he sees it, it's only a positive. (At $6,000 a pop, of course it is.) "Even if some of the kids are ultimately not successful, at least when they come here they're happy," he says. "It's a happy place. And they have a reprieve."

He takes great pride in the camp's "Commitment to Care," its human rights statement that each kid must sign upon arrival. He waves it in the air. "I try to inculcate [into] the kids that we need each and every one of them to accept each other, to say hello to each other, to include them in their games, to talk to somebody if they're sad—just to help each other," he says. "The idea is for the campers themselves to create a community where anyone that comes in is included and part of it and they are all friendly and we don't care what you look like. You need to be able to like yourself no matter what you look like, because you may never get that body."

It's an excellent plan, a utopian ideal. If only it worked. But actually, what they look like *is* a problem; the whole goal is to change their appearance. And let's be honest, if he really believed that, the camp wouldn't exist.

And, of course, bullying goes on, despite the piece of paper. It's naïve to think it wouldn't.

"The people were still being made fun of about their weight," says Rebecca Donaldson, fifteen, who has spent three summers at Shane. "The more overweight kids are still made fun of."

Like Tony Sparber—the two men are deeply competitive—Ettenberg believes that parents contribute to the problem. (Even Ben Weill's mother told me they used to go out for dim sum the night before they took him to camp.) Genetics play a role, too. Still, he says, "At some point kids need to be responsible for their own behavior. Everybody is quick to blame somebody else."

After the summer he offers Camp Shane at Home, where he works with 300 nutritionists around the country. (What about kids who don't live there, I wonder? What do they do?) He says he pays part of the bill and encourages families to see a nutritionist. "Instead of fighting with their kids we really encourage families to find a registered dietitian to do the fighting," he says. "They might need therapy, too. It all depends. Don't forget, we're dealing with a wide spectrum of kids. You've got kids here who sometimes have no emotional problems or behavioral problems, they just have poor eating habits. They're just eating too much."

Camp, he says, is a little like rehab. "Call it what you want—education, cold turkey—there's no alternative here. You don't have to fight your temptations. You can't do 'should I or shouldn't I' because there's no possibility. You're forced to eat properly. Before they come to camp a lot of the kids don't know anything about nutrition. Do they truly know what calories mean? Do they know portion size? Even recipes—four ounces of this, three ounces of that—what does that mean? You grow up and you're a little kid and you get served portions at every meal. You get into bad eating habits right away in this country. Nobody has a cooking scale at home. But you come to camp and you start seeing what the portions look like and that's educational in itself."

"It's really an awesome camp, period," he continues. "We don't focus on weight. This is a camp so there is singing and dancing and playing and everyone's just having a grand old time. We're not walking around saying, 'We're overweight.' It's not a depressed place. It's a happy place."

» «

That might be true for many, but it's not to Lucy Walker and Sarah Carter, two of Shane's so-called guidance counselors. In the real world Carter is a social worker in her native Yorkshire, England; Walker is a registered nurse from Omaha, Nebraska, who teaches high school health.

Most camps offer some kind of quasi group therapy, when the kids are supposed to talk about their weight-related issues in the supportive and understanding environment they lack elsewhere. When I was a camper, we would meet twice a week, ostensibly to discuss our feelings about weight. But invariably the conversation would devolve into an in-depth exploration into bunk dynamics or why we weren't cleaning up after ourselves. The weight became an afterthought—not an entirely bad thing, since it gave us a chance to be normal kids with normal problems. On the other hand, we never really looked at our issues, which we desperately needed to do.

Camp Kingsmont, which was in the Berkshires and is now on the Hampshire College campus in Northampton, Massachusetts, calls its counseling program Connections; Tony Sparber's Camp Pocono Trails calls it Be Your Best!; and Camp La Jolla, in California, dubs it B-Mod (short for behavior modification). At Shane it goes by "rap" and is often led by a nurse, nutritionist, or, if no one better is around, a counselor. The goal is to give campers skills and information they can use when they return home: nutritional information, portion control, the ability to recognize why they eat when they don't really want to.

Generally speaking, the girls get into rap much more than the guys do. (Ben Weill says it's "forty minutes when you don't have to run.")

On this day, a humid afternoon in mid-July, twenty-eight girls ages eleven to thirteen sit in a circle in a wooden gazebo at Camp Shane. The gazebo is all the way at the bottom of a 90-degree hill that the kids must climb at least six times a day. (The dining hall is at the bottom, and God knows they want to eat.) They look like typical preteens: floppy hats, T-shirts, jeans, flip-flops. Acne. Braces. They don't look that big to me, but then, most have been here for six weeks already.

Sarah Carter, who reminds me of Jane Leeves from *Frasier*, leads today's conversation. A tiny wisp of a thing with big blue eyes, short auburn hair, and freckles dotting her face, she is in her early twenties and the kids seem to relate well to her. Since she's a social worker, she actually has somewhat of a clue what she's talking about. I have high hopes for this meeting; maybe they will actually discuss something useful, and reach some level of insight into their problems.

Sarah stands before the girls, clutching a clipboard. "Some people are very worried about leaving camp," she says. "What are some of your worries?"

The girls raise their hands.

"I'm worried that I'm going to gain the weight back or I'm not going to stick to the diet," says Heather.

"I'm worried that my parents won't encourage me," says Vanessa.

Another girl, Lisa, divides her time between her dad's house and her mom's, and it's confusing. "My dad and my stepmom are a lot of help; he comes home and makes grilled chicken. The problem is that my stepdad and mom eat different foods."

Sarah nods sympathetically. This is a common problem; parents really aren't as supportive as they should be. They think the child's weight issues have disappeared just because he's thinner. They're wrong.

"We go to my grandmother's house once a week, and I'm worried I'm going to have trouble with portions," says Kerry.

"One of my problems is that after camp, me, my brother, my dad, and my stepmom fly to Florida and visit some family and stay there for a while, and then from Florida we go to an island for vacation and there's a lot of fattening foods," says Kristin. "My first time doing this was last summer—we went to Aruba. This summer we're going on a cruise for a week. There's a lot of food on these cruises." (No kidding! Why would her parents subject her to that?)

"When you leave the camp your parents get a lovely little pack about that thick"—Sarah indicates size with her thumb and forefinger—"and there's a booklet with handy tips about what to do when you get home and go to restaurants and things like that," she says. "Parents are genuinely lost when it comes to this stuff. People who have never had a weight issue, it's really hard for them to get their head around the fact that they've got to start thinking about these things. You've done all this hard work and you don't want it to go to waste."

A girl named Hannah laughs. "I have chocolate in front of me and I see it and all I can think of is, 'Big bar of chocolate there, big bar of chocolate there!'"

Everyone howls. But then Leigh speaks up and the girls get quiet again.

"Before I left for camp my mother said to me—'please lose weight.'" She starts to cry, and the girl next to her rubs her back.

"Parents love their children but they don't know how to handle weight issues," Sarah says gently.

Now the girls start shouting things out:

"At my school you're allowed to go up and get seconds and the food is real greasy. I'm bigger than everyone and I get made fun of a lot," says Karen. "Most people aren't nice if you're overweight."

"I'll ask my mom for guidance," says Rose. "But she was never overweight. She's skinny and it bothers me."

"I know my parents care, but like other people say, I came here to learn how to live a lifestyle to stay healthy. But what I'm worried about is going home and having them think I can do it myself," Randy says.

Finally one girl looks on the bright side: "Being fat has its advantage, because I can easily body slam these teenagers who make fun of me!" Applause and hoots all around.

» «

Now it's the boys' turn. They're much less effusive than the girls; they fidget and poke at each other and Sarah has to reprimand them constantly. Still, they make some pretty revealing statements.

"What I'm asking for is that we listen, we speak individually, we have no swinging out on the gazebo, and we listen," says Sarah. "So what I want to talk about are the fears you might have about leaving camp and about when you get home."

Ten-year-old Jordan pipes up at once. "One of my fears about leaving camp is that when I get home I can't seem to lose weight because there's no way you can get anywhere close to the food we eat here," he says. "At home you can just open the cabinets, but here there are no cabinets. You have nowhere to go for food. It's hard at home because food is always in my cabinets."

"So you're worried that when you're at home if there is food in the cabinet you're more likely to eat it? That's a good one," says Sarah. "What we're talking about is willpower. Portion control. You can eat junk food sometimes. But you have to make the right choices the rest of the time."

"I'm gonna put a lock on my cabinet," says Zach, twelve.

"I'm not really scared about eating so much because I'm so young," says twelve-year-old Jess. "I'll just have to learn how to slow it down. I'm gonna do Weight Watchers at home. Since I'm so young I get thirty points."

"I'm worried that when I get home I'm going to be tempted to eat the wrong foods," says Michael, ten. "Here they don't have fast foods and we have fast foods at our house."

Max, eleven, is totally hyperactive; he simply can't sit still. "I just eat way too much at home," he says. "I can never fall asleep at night without eating something. I keep getting bigger. I always sneak a sandwich at night."

"What I'm actually worried about is gaining the weight back," says Jake, eleven. "Sometimes when I'm bored I'll just go upstairs and I'll open the cabinet and I'll eat something. Or like sometimes my mom will make a separate plate for me and then my sister and my mom and dad will eat the regular meal and I'll go eat it later on."

"I gotta get active," says Ron, ten. "I sit in my basement and do nothing."

"I sit in front of the television for hours and hours. I spend from, like, six o'clock in the morning on a normal Saturday watching TV," says Alex, eleven.

"You have to build a snowman," Jake offers.

"I'm worried about going home and gaining weight," says an eight-year-old kid, Adam—one of only four black kids I have seen. "I weigh more than my brother—I'm really ashamed of it."

"Oh yeah—none of my friends know this is a fat camp," says

Max. "I never told them it was a fat camp. I just told them it was an active camp."

"I'm proud," says Jess. "I told my friends."

"I told them where I was going, too," says Zack. "And about all the fun."

"Some people are not the most supportive," says Sarah. She does not offer any solutions—and really, what is there to say? Oh, she could offer the usual words of encouragement: That after working so hard and achieving so much it would be a shame to blow it; that nothing tastes as good as thin feels; that this is the first day of the rest of their lives, blah blah blah. But the truth is the kids probably *will* gain back their weight, and their parents probably *won't* understand how they feel, and their friends *will* wonder how they got so thin, and then why they're getting so big again. Sure, she could tell them that camp is only the beginning of a never-ending struggle that will most likely cause them despair until they finally somehow decide not to let it, but why be so bleak?

Besides, it's time for a snack.

» «

After the kids leave for their next activity, I hang around for a post-mortem with Sarah, who's absolutely wiped out. She's just led two rap sessions, and spent another twenty minutes consoling a despondent camper. Hers is a twenty-hour-a-day job and frankly, not worth the money.

"This is my first time in the U.S. and I can understand why kids are so fat. You go into McDonald's and it's refills, refills, refills, and all you can eat," she says.

"Would you come back to camp?" I ask.

She sighs. "I think that Camp Shane can offer a great jump start for some of the children that are dangerously overweight; it offers a controlled environment where the child will almost definitely lose weight and it gets them to think about what they are eating and a chance to talk to other children in the same situation," she says.

"However, with all diets, if the person does not recognize there is a problem and is not committed to change and it's forced upon them then I think it is a waste of time. I can only imagine that for some children this will cause relationship problems with the parents and possibly a future lack of trust."

She says that she thinks the camp only offers a temporary solution, and that the diet is "unrealistic," causing an unhealthy focus on food. At one point she asked the kids what they would be doing when they got home. Almost all replied: "All-you-can-eat Chinese buffet!" or "McDonald's!"

(I ask Emily Williams, who went to Camp Kingsmont, if the focus on food is a problem. "Yeah," she says. "It makes me feel deprived."

On one field trip to the Six Flags amusement park, she tells me she ate chicken fingers, French fries, a hot dog. "How'd you feel after?" I asked.

"Not bad," she shrugged. "It was like, 'I want more.'")

"Kids need to learn that they can eat what they want but in proportion—and with exercise," Sarah continues. "Also, they need to taste nice low-fat/healthy foods so that they will be encouraged to eat more of them. The meals at Shane are not something that as a child I would have tried to cook or asked my mother to buy for me. The camp needs to look at this.

"It's also an unnatural environment," she adds. "When the kids go back home or school they won't be able to do six one-hour activities. They will have to develop their own idea of what is a reasonable amount of exercise to do in a week to help keep up a healthy lifestyle."

Her biggest peeve is that there are so many thin kids at camp with distorted body images. "The issues that are faced by the overweight child are different from the issues faced by a child who is pencil-thin and thinks that she's overweight," she says. "This can send out very dangerous messages if the two are mixed."

She also believes the staff should be knowledgeable about—or at least interested in—weight loss and kids, and not there for their own weight loss agendas. I agree with this wholeheartedly. When I was at camp we would have the occasional counselor with a psycho-logical interest in kids and weight-related issues, or a nutrition major earning college credit, but they were anomalies.

Fran Moscowitz, a mom from Baltimore, sent her daughter, Ilana, to Shane in the summer of 2003. Moscowitz is irate that she didn't receive any professional assessment of her daughter's progress. "They don't give a report back—nothing geared toward my kid," says Moscowitz angrily. "When I sent my dog to the kennel camp, I got a report card back."

As for Sarah, she doesn't plan to return to Shane, although maybe she should. By camp's end, she has put on fourteen pounds.

» «

One important point Sarah makes is that successful weight loss involves the entire family. For a child to truly lose weight, the whole clan needs to stand behind her. This can be daunting, especially if there are other members in the family who can eat whatever they want. Doesn't matter. You can't buy treats for your skinny child while forbidding your overweight kid from eating them. The entire household *has* to embrace the bigger child's efforts.

Parents need to use common sense. If young Jake has just returned from three or six or eight weeks in an environment where he cannot eat whatever he wants, where his meals are regulated and his portions controlled, then there's a good chance he'll be pretty freaked out about food when he gets into the real world. He might not trust himself to stay on track; he might not even know what to eat. Or, conversely, he might know what he *should* eat but because of the deprivation he's experienced all summer, he'll go right for the bad stuff. It may sound surprising, but lots of parents don't know that they shouldn't keep junk food in the house—even if they have other children who aren't heavy. Or that they themselves shouldn't eat junk in front of their kids. Or that they should encourage their kids to exercise. Or that they shouldn't be afraid to set down rules

37

on TV and computer use. After spending all this money, parents have to be present. They have to be, well, parents.

If this seems obvious, just talk to Lydia Burton, who spent two summers working at a weight loss camp. At the time, Burton, now twenty-four, was looking to do something between college and grad school. She was hired as a counselor but since she had studied psychology, she found herself acting as camp shrink. She returned her second year as a guidance counselor, and boy did she get an eyeful.

"It's a sad statement, but I feel the majority of parents would rather give their kids a pill than pick them up and be involved in some way," says Lydia. "You saw some awful parenting at camp and parents aren't required to do anything. They can send the kids off and do nothing else. A lot of these parents just want to get rid of their child for the summer. A lot don't come on visiting day. There are seminars for parents, but a lot of parents don't show up, so the kids go back to the exact same situations. They learn a little bit at camp, but the parents still continue to feed them the way they have been. After camp ends the child either gains it back or the kid leaves with an intense fear of food. A couple have told me that they're afraid of food and they're terrified of overeating, of portions. They say, 'I can't think of food normally anymore.' It's a borderline eating disorder."

Two summers ago Burton had a camper from Beverly Hills, "sweet as could be, not heavy at all, worked her ass off, took all the hard classes," she recalls. "Her mom was calling her counselor weekly. She was upset because her daughter was gaining muscle when she was just supposed to lose weight. 'I want her on a stricter diet,' she said. We were like, 'Absolutely not.' When the mother came to pick her up, in front of everyone, kids and counselors, she said, 'I'm so disappointed in you! You didn't lose weight! You thought fat camp was hard? Wait till you get home to Camp Mommy. One meal a day.' Social services weren't called, but they should have been. The kid just smirked and walked away with her mom.

"There were kids who probably should have been at an institution, not at a weight-loss camp," she says. "There were some very disturbed kids, and weight was secondary. A couple of times I said to the director, 'We're not equipped to deal with this type of situation—we're not a mental health facility.' The majority of the kids were compulsive overeaters, which is why they were there. And a lot were medicated and had experienced horrific life events: sexual abuse, the death of a parent. When I was a counselor there, four out of my eight girls had lost a parent. They were thirteen years old and could trace the weight gain back to that.

"The problem with a lot of these kids is they are so active here while they are at camp and then they go home to PlayStation or the computer or something and that's the end of their physical exercise," she continues. "It's hard for a lot of these kids because you know a lot of them are not going to leave camp at the weight they want to be. That's just a given. So they come home still overweight and they don't want to get involved in sports and they don't want to get involved in that kind of stuff at school, and I think that is why it's so hard. You really need that to be able to keep the weight off, yet because of the fact that you're overweight you're intimidated to do that kind of stuff. It's a really hard situation."

And their problems weren't manifested in weight alone. Burton saw a lot of cutting and self-mutilation. "I worked very intensely with one camper who was only allowed to stay on the basis that she not cut herself. She had been hospitalized and diagnosed with borderline personality disorder. She took meds. Mind you, I should never have been trying to intervene with these kids—I'm not a psychologist, I'd just earned my master's! We always had someone on call; we had kids threatening to jump out of the window in the middle of the night. We'd try to talk them down. This summer I was so stressed out I ate a lot of candy, I'd stay in my apartment eating, watching TV, wishing I wasn't there."

Savvy camps know that parents are usually in need of help, too, and over the past few years programs for the entire family have sprung up at camps (La Jolla), spas (Canyon Ranch), and medical weight-loss facilities (Pritikin Longevity Center and Spa, Duke University). They're all variations on the same theme: eating healthy, exercising, trying to educate kids and parents on the importance of healthy eating and exercising. But they're not cheap. Two weeks at Pritikin, in Turnberry Isle, Florida, costs $7,732 ($8,232 in the winter months). A summer at La Jolla runs about $9,000 a person. Clearly, not every parent can afford places like this.

Mary Stevens is one of the lucky ones. Forty-seven years old, she's the mother of two—one son, George, who is a super jock, and Andrew, who is not as athletically inclined. Stevens, who's currently not working (her husband owns a printing company), went to Camp La Jolla two years in a row with Andrew, who is now fourteen. When she arrived, she weighed 192 at five foot two; her son was 235. They lived in separate areas of the campus—he with kids his age, she with older women and other mothers. It was the best summer of their lives.

"I didn't want my son to feel as if my husband and I were sending him away because something was wrong," she says, explaining why she decided to join Andrew at La Jolla (that, and the fact that she was also obese).

"I wasn't quite sure what I was getting into. I understand from the literature this is not a therapeutic community, it's not psychologically based, it's not like there are weight-management specialists who were going to pick his brain and show him the underlying psychological basis of his eating. It's more weight loss from behavior modification and nutritional education."

Originally they only planned to stay for four weeks, but they did so well they stayed for nine. She lost thirty-eight pounds and her son lost forty-seven. They returned the following summer having only gained about fifteen pounds—a relative success story.

"It's become a family affair with us," she says. "We were at the gym Monday through Thursday from 4 to 5:15 P.M. I'm convinced we kept off the majority of the weight because we incorporated exercise into our lifestyle. There is a lot of dysfunction in every family and I think my family has a share and that needs to be addressed for me and Andrew to remain successful. I also believe that the mother is extremely important in the family dynamic. Not that the father isn't, but for Andrew and me it's a lifelong process and that's what I had to get in my head and his head. This is not a diet, this is just a lifestyle change and I think that's so important."

Mary and Andrew *are* success stories. Still, that doesn't mean that they didn't have setbacks. Her older son, George, the athlete, doesn't have a weight problem. Neither does her husband. She admits that she allowed herself to be swayed by their needs. "I felt bad. At one point George started yelling at me, 'How come we never have any snacks, Mom?' So I go buy this whole bag full of stuff and hide it. I'm not doing that anymore. George and my husband can go outside the house and get their Dairy Queens and their candy bars."

» «

Lucy Walker spent the summer of 2003 at Camp Shane with her sixteen-year-old daughter, Blythe. Shane doesn't have a family program, but Blythe wanted to lose weight and rather than send her off by herself, Walker, forty-two, decided to go with her and became a counselor. After it was clear that she was older and more experienced than the average counselor, she was promoted to guidance counselor.

At first, the beauty of Camp Shane overwhelmed her. Such big weight loss! Such acceptance! She's been married to her high-school sweetheart for twenty-one years and has two kids. She has big blue eyes, Cover Girl skin, and a flat Midwestern accent. She also possesses—or did, anyway—the misguided belief that things really are the way they seem to be. She hoped to get a free summer for her daughter, but that didn't quite happen: "I got a tuition break, but I still gave David a healthy check. And I worked my ass off—twenty hours a day." She also lived in a cabin with thirteen-year-old girls, which she'd never done before—even when she herself was thirteen.

"This is my first time and it's been amazing," she says. "The kids look so different. You have to do a double take and wonder, 'Is that who I think it is?' because they no longer look how they used to look. I thought I was doing life-changing work back home—no, this is life-changing work. I get hugs like you wouldn't believe.

"I had no clue they would come with such baggage—ADD [Attention Deficit Disorder], Asperger's," she continues. "If they have an eating disorder we recognize it and they're sent home, because we don't have the psychotherapy sessions to deal with eating disorders here. But many of the parents are the problems themselves. We had another girl whose mother came on visiting day and said, 'I thought by now you'd be a size 0.' The next day the girl wouldn't eat at all. And we wonder why the kids are doing this. We're doing it to them."

Fair enough. But look, I point out, you're a mom—and you think of yourself as a good one—you're happily married, and yet your daughter has a food and weight problem. What's that about?

Walker sighs and explains that her daughter was always shy and never felt like she fit in anywhere. So she self-medicated with food. She also takes after her father, who is six feet tall and large-boned. (Walker is about five foot one and has never had a weight problem.)

"As a nurse, I was afraid of saying anything because I was afraid I would push her into the eating disorders," she says. "Look at our media, look what it does to women in particular. Look at *American Idol.* In one segment you had the young lady from Georgia who was kicked out because she was too chunky. Simon chewed her up and spit her out and yet who was the one that won? Wasn't it Ruben, the very large African American man who they call the Teddy Bear? It was not okay for the women to be heavy but perfectly fine for the men. We do that to our children."

Instead of mentioning her daughter's weight, she never brought it up at all. It simply didn't exist. But then Blythe saw the MTV special about Shane and asked her mom if she could go. "I gave up my life to come here," says Walker, not unkindly. "Anything that would make her happy I'm more than willing to do, but kids should come with instructions. If I had known then what I know now I would have really made sure that I did the portion-control stuff and that you were only allowed to eat at meals and only in the kitchen. We lived that typical life with fast food because I'm a working mom. If it was a bad day for me they were lucky they ate, and I allowed them to sit and watch TV and chew on whatever they wanted to in the evenings. We drank our calories. Those were the unhappy lifestyle things that we did. Is that going to change now? Oh, yeah."

» «

On her way back from camp—Blythe thirty pounds lighter, her mother six pounds heavier—Lucy had an Epiphanic Moment: *I'll start my own camp! I'll do it myself! And better!*

She and Blythe discussed this all the way home, through the flat-lands and fields of Ohio, Indiana, and Illinois, and she asked God for a sign. When she got home the lead story on the news that night was that nationally one in seven kids is obese. That was enough for her.

She immediately kicked into gear, finding land in the Midwest and taking out a bank loan. No, she had no business background—she didn't understand all the legal stuff and insurance and such—but she was trainable.

"What I learned is that camp is really big business," she says. But her camp—Camp Slim Summer (not its real name)—wouldn't be about dollars. It would genuinely be about making a difference. "I can say that my heart's in the right spot. I look at the kids and they're very needy and we need to do a lot of work with them. I hope to have campers come back and show me how good they're doing."

To do this, she created a plan from scratch. For one thing, there would be a salad bar with real lettuce, not the nonnutritious iceberg found at Shane. She would hold nutrition and behavior-modifica-tion classes twice a week. Four weeks would cost $3,190 per camper, but her hope was to target lower- and middle-class kids and offer scholarships. She even set up an advisory board comprised of Wash-ington University medical staff.

There would be one eight-week session or two four-week ses-sions; camp would offer horseback riding, rock climbing, hiking, and, of course, fitness classes. Those who stayed the second session would take on some kind of leadership role. "Eight weeks is enough, and I'm not trying to steal people's money," she says. "Let's give it to them in four weeks. If kids stay longer because they have more weight to lose, now let's build self-esteem. I only want the kids to come for one summer. If they come back the second year I know it didn't work and I'll just be taking their money." Camp Slim Summer is now looking forward to its second season.

» «

Some parents, like Kevin Marema's, recognize that camp is a short-lived panacea that generally fails in the long term. Kevin, who's now twelve, spent one summer at Tony Sparber's Florida camp and two summers at Camp La Jolla. He has seen two different dietitians, worked out with a personal trainer, done Pilates with his mom, tried the South Beach Diet, and visited a pediatric gastroenterologist who specialized in childhood obesity. Whatever weight he lost, he quickly regained.

When he was ten, five feet tall and nearly 200 pounds, his parents, Rita and Robert, flew him to Mexico to have a balloon inserted in his stomach. Both Rita and Robert—a gastric bypass surgeon in Fort Lauderdale—had undergone gastric bypass surgery and thought that might help their son. Although the device—its proper name is bariatric intragastric balloon (BIB)—is not approved in the United States, the procedure is less invasive than gastric bypass. A balloon is put into the stomach and inflated, giving one the feeling of being full, and thereby diminishing the desire to eat.

Kevin hated it. He could feel the balloon pressing against his insides when he moved, and he only lost fifteen pounds, which he promptly regained when the balloon was removed nine months later.

After the failed balloon experiment, his parents offered him gastric bypass surgery—he would have been the youngest person in this country to get it—but he declined.

"He said, 'Mommy, I'm only twelve!'" Rita Marema recalls. In the spring of 2004, a family friend told him about a boarding school for overweight kids, called the Academy of the Sierras (AOS). Kevin immediately went to the Web site.

"I knew it was one of my only choices," says Kevin, who is bright and articulate, with a cherubic face and big brown eyes. "I wasn't doing well after two months at a weight-loss camp. I was gaining back my weight plus some, and I just felt this was almost my last resort until surgery."

On many levels Kevin is a typical preteen. He loves his iPod and Bose headphones. He's crazy about PlayStations. But his true passion, his life's calling, is Walt Disney. He owns dozens of Mickey and Donald and Goofy shirts and DVDs and posters and figurines. He has collected over 500 Disney pins. His favorite channel is—yes—Disney. His goal is to sit on the Disney board. He has been to Disney World more times than he can count.

"It's a place where I can just relax," he says, sounding older than his twelve years. "I go there and I don't think about anything else. I just go and have fun. Everyone has a place to go and forget about things, and that's my place."

He needed it. In December 2003, the family moved into a sparkling new two-story Mediterranean-style home in Fort Lauderdale, right at the edge of a canal. Three weeks later Kevin's father moved out and filed for divorce. Rita was devastated; Kevin gained fifty pounds, his weight shooting up to 240 within six months.

"Kevin has always had a weight problem—he weighed ten pounds, three ounces at birth, two weeks early," Rita, fifty-one, says with a laugh. But this was the heaviest her son had ever been, and she was truly at a loss.

Although Rita knows Kevin's weight problems are largely the result of genetics—the propensity for weight gain is simply in his DNA—she blames herself.

"I decided not to monitor what Kevin ate when he was growing up," she says. "You read all the books and you want to do everything the right way, and they tell you not to do that. So, I wouldn't hide anything, I wouldn't limit anything. But I remember bringing a bag of Goldfish to a party at his school, and all the kids would take one at a time, and he would take a handful." If she had to do it over again she would have never taken him out for fast food. She would have cooked nutritious meals that they ate together as a family.

Kevin thinks that's ridiculous. "I knew even at nine that I had a weight problem and that fast food wouldn't have done any good for me. I feel like I should have been responsible for myself. I should have made better choices than three Happy Meals."

In September 2004, Kevin became one of twelve students at AOS. The school is run by Ryan Craig, a Toronto-born, Yale-educated lawyer. Craig, thirty-four, spent three years as a vice president at Warburg-Pincus, the international private equity firm in Manhattan, where he ran their education and training division. As soon as he arrived at Warburg he began researching investment options for them; one in particular, called Aspen Education, caught his eye. Headquartered in Cerritos, California, Aspen operates forty-one "therapeutic intervention" programs in thirteen states, including long-term residential, outpatient services, special-education day schools, and outdoor therapy and wilderness programs for kids with behavioral and substance abuse problems. About 50,000 adolescents have gone through the various programs; unfortunately, there are no official statistics, although Craig says they have about a 90 percent success rate (that is, students who stay sober or alcohol-free).

From the moment Craig got involved with Aspen—he's a former board member—he wondered whether it might be wise for them to tackle childhood obesity. He'd heard the statistics and wondered why there weren't any longer term residential facilities for this population.

He immersed himself in the field, and soon came to the conclusion that nobody was really doing it right. He thought he could figure out how, or at least make inroads. So why not just do it himself?

"A number of people at Warburg told me I was crazy; I could have stayed there and made a lot of money," says Craig, a tall, angular man with a quirky sense of humor, who has never had a weight problem and likely never will. Nor has anyone in his family. Still, the subject spoke to him. He feels for both the overweight children and their parents, who are often exasperated and utterly befuddled by their child's problem.

"Most of these kids have inherited a biology which makes it very easy for them to gain weight and even harder for them to lose it," Craig says. "And I think parents feel a lot of shame around this."

I first met Craig in November 2002, after he read an online posting of mine. He e-mailed me and asked what I thought about a boarding school for overweight kids, if I thought parents would be willing to pay $5,500 a month to send their child off to learn and lose weight. The schools he had in mind would be called Healthy Living Academies—not Fat Schools—and would offer physical and psychological therapy, nutrition and cooking classes, and lectures on healthy living, in addition to a traditional curriculum that was tailored for each student. Credits would be transferable and recognized by colleges. The by-product, hopefully, would be a shedding of their sedentary, calorie-rich lifestyles in favor of healthier ones.

"My hypothesis is that a residential school environment would be the optimal environment to address weight issues for many teens," he wrote in his e-mail. "On the other hand, perhaps such an environment wouldn't be ideal in that it would reinforce the child's identity as overweight or obese."

I thought it was a great idea—sort of. I would have given anything to spend a year slimming down away from home. A boarding school would have been beyond my wildest dreams, and I searched high and low for a place, but never found one. That's because it didn't exist. (Actually, there is a program in Germany, called the Insula Rehabilitation Centre, which has been around for twelve years and is run by the Protestant Church of Bavaria. It's a complex of several units—a kindergarten, a home for the elderly, a children's preschool, and the Obesity Rehabilitation Center, a treatment facility for adolescents aged thirteen and up. Most stay about six months—they go to school, do therapy, exercise, and hopefully learn techniques to keep weight off. Unlike AOS, it is covered by health insurance.)

But I had concerns. For one thing, the school would cost over $5,500 a month—roughly the same price as, say, a high-end boarding school like Andover or Choate. This doesn't really help the lower classes, who have the highest rates of obesity. It wouldn't even help for the middle class.

"If they can afford to send their kids to college, many middle-class families should be able to afford a semester or two at one of our schools," Craig said. When I pointed out that many families can't afford $50,000 a year precisely because they are saving for college, he said, "You're right. But in many cases if you don't get treatment now, they won't be going to college. Studies are reporting increased rates of depression, low self-esteem, and social isolation with overweight kids, which are then manifested in significant behavioral problems. As these children grow up, they're less likely to be accepted into college, less likely to get married, and more likely to occupy a lower socioeconomic status." (Fair enough. It still doesn't mean their parents can afford AOS.)

Mostly, I worried about the kids themselves. Would they feel that they were being shipped off as punishment because they were fat? Did they really need to be isolated and segregated from the rest of the world?

Ryan Craig had tossed all of these questions around in his head, and ultimately decided that the benefits outweighed the potential pitfalls. This would be a different model from the regular weight-loss camp, something revolutionary in the United States.

In January 2003, he quit his job at Warburg, moved to Santa Monica, where his wife, Yahlin Chang, a writer for *ER*, was living, and devoted himself full time to Healthy Living Academies.

To do it right, he assembled a group of high-level players in the obesity field to sit on the school's advisory board, including Dr. Kelly D. Brownell, director of the Yale Center for Eating and Weight Disorders. He hired Dr. Daniel Kirschenbaum, professor of psychiatry and behavioral sciences at Northwestern University Medical School, in Chicago, as the clinical director. He found a place in Reedley, California, the site of a former Aspen school that had recently closed (before that it was a psychiatric hospital). He had no students, but that didn't worry him. He would build it, and they would come.

During the same time period, he developed two Aspen-run weight-loss summer camps: Camp Wellspring, an all-girl camp in the Adirondacks, and Camp Wellspring Adventure, in the mountains of North Carolina, a sort of Outward Bound for overweight kids. By June 2003, both were up and running with about fifty campers each, some of whom he hoped would continue on at the school. These camps differed from the more traditional weight-loss camps in that they offered a clinical program developed by Dr. Kirschenbaum and the advisory board.

For starters, every camper monitored his or her own eating, jotting down the foods, calories, and fat grams in a little journal. (They were supposed to eat 20 grams of fat per day, and about 1,200 calories.) They were given pedometers and aimed for at least 10,000 steps a day. Most important, *they* regulated their food intake, not a counselor—an important distinction.

At meals, for example, campers were offered "at will," or uncontrolled, foods, like berries, melons, or fat-free soups. They were free to eat as much of those as they wanted. "They can eat 3,000 calories a day if they want," says Kirschenbaum. "Our hope is that they're going to choose to regulate it."

Kirschenbaum, fifty-one, believes self-control can be taught like any other skill—playing the cello, say, or riding a bike—through instruction, modeling, and encouragement. "Self-control is a process in behavioral terms, keeping track of target behaviors and systematically evaluating these behaviors, goal-setting. When they write down what they're eating, that's self-control."

"But how do you know that they're not lying?" I ask.

"If they're going to go through the trouble of getting weighed in and the parents are involved, what would be the point? The main purpose of self-monitoring is not just information. When you write something down you're thinking about what you're trying to do. So we encourage people to concentrate on goals they believe are important in their lives no matter what's going on. We're trying to get them to truly obsess in a positive way, so they feel bad if they don't exercise or eat healthy."

Kirshenbaum and Craig also held a parent workshop at the end of each camp session, to educate parents on what their children were going through. Although most camps offer some kind of parental lecture, only a handful of adults actually show up, and the sessions only scratch the surface. It's a two-day affair at the Wellspring Camps, even though only about twenty sets of parents came for the workshop in July, and only five in August. Parents were handed their own pedometers and self-monitoring journals and were told to walk in their kids' shoes for a day. "We talk a lot about how they're going to need to live it in order to promote this change in their kids," says Craig.

Craig built a three-month after-care program into the cost of the camp ($3,800 for one month; $6,800 for two), which included an online diary where students could list their activity levels and food choices. Wellspring counselors communicated with kids and tracked their progress via e-mail and phone. About a third of the campers—about forty kids—participated in the After-Care program with the level of consistency necessary to be a successful long-term weight controller. Of these, none reported any weight gain during the three-month after-care program; some maintained, and a few continued to lose weight. (One camper lost nearly thirty pounds over the summer and then went on to lose another thirty pounds over the following three months. But she was a rarity.)

By summer's end, three campers signed on for the boarding school; another eleven, who had heard about it from nutritionists or doctors, had also enrolled. By September, the first students arrived at the Academy of the Sierras, pioneers in the war against weight. Kevin Marema was one of them.

» «

The Academy of the Sierras sits on sixty-eight acres in the San Joaquin Valley, about twenty-five miles southeast of Fresno, California. This is farm country, a land of raisins and peaches, where trac-tors seemingly outnumber Toyotas. The day I visit is bone-dry, the sun slanting over the fruit fields. I pass students running, walking, or bike riding on a dirt road outside of the school, part of their daily routine.

Each morning before breakfast, students must either walk, bike, or take an aerobic class, the first of their two daily organized physi-cal activities. (A typical day starts at 7 A.M. and ends at 10 P.M., with lights out by 11.) Craig is right there with them, working up a sweat.

The kids look like kids everywhere, with multiple piercings, tat-toos, pimples. They are bigger, certainly, and they move slower, per-haps, but the banter between them is no different from other high school kids. Between classes, some lose themselves in their iPods; others jabber away. They range in age from twelve to twenty, with a few more girls than boys; the average weight hovers around 230 pounds (the heaviest arrived at over 500).

Teenagers in general are often depressed and angry, but AOS stu-dents have the added burden of being large in a cruel and unforgiv-ing world. Many are medicated and treated for depression, although none have any major health problems (yet). Whether their obesity contributes to their depression or is the result of it is some-what irrelevant; by the time they come to school the two are indeli-bly intertwined. Still, on the surface, the AOS students don't seem especially troubled. Rather, they seem happy to be here, as if they know they're doing something positive for themselves.

"These kids aren't as hostile and angry as the kids at other Aspen Education programs," says residential director Dan Barry, thirty, who has been working at Aspen for five years. "These kids *want* to be here, which makes all the difference in the world."

Not that they don't complain. They do, big time. They're home-sick, they're tired, they're only allowed to make two phone calls a week. *It's not fair!* They want their cell phones, which were confis-cated when they arrived.

"I was completely pissed off about that for a week and a half," says Daniel Burger, a sixteen-year-old from Phoenix.

"It's just not right!" echoes Natasha Ulch, fifteen, twirling a small silver tongue ring. "I need to talk to my friends at home."

They do have a chance to get their cell phones back. They just have to earn the right to use them. The school operates on a Summit System, a five-tiered reward system designed to motivate kids. New students, for example, are called Gumbies. To move up to the next rung, they must average 10,000 steps for two weeks in a row, complete their food log twenty out of thirty-six meals, meet their academic goals, and clean their rooms and community areas. After two weeks, they can apply for Boulderer status, which gives them, among other privileges, a chance to go to a movie once a week. By the time they reach the fifth level—about six months—Yabo (named for California mountain climber John Yablonsky), they will have demonstrated sufficient self-control and earned the right to design their own program. As Yabos, they're given junior staff responsibilities, and could, conceivably, get their cell phones back.

Three times a day—four, counting snack—students hurry into the cafeteria, their pedometers clipped to their belt loops or waistbands. The place looks like any school lunchroom, except for the blackboard with words of encouragement scribbled on it ("Self-monitoring is the path to success!"), and the total number of calories, protein, and fat grams, which are also listed next to each food item. There are controlled and uncontrolled foods. Students can have as much of the latter as they wish; the idea is for them to take responsibility for their choices.

And they do. They come to the meals with their Calorie Counter and minijournals, and talk about the meal in their own special language, a shorthand unique to them.

"How much is in the scrambled eggs? Sixty calories and twelve grams of protein?" asks Kevin Marema, straining his neck to read the blackboard. He scribbles in his journal. "That's low."

Almost all of them drink Diet Coke or Diet Sprite with every meal, even breakfast. This is the least of Craig's concerns. He operates under the principle of least intervention, which is why students are allowed as much artificial sweetener, caffeine, salt, or soy sauce as they want. (Kevin's favorite is soy sauce, which he slathers over everything. He even calls himself Soy Boy.)

"We can't control them," says Craig. "If they want to drink Diet Coke for breakfast, go for it."

Students meet with a therapist, or behavioral coach, four to seven times a week, both one-on-one and in a group setting. The assistant clinical director is Molly Carmel, twenty-seven, who sees every single student at least once a week.

An MSW and former counselor at Phoenix House, a drug rehabilitation center in Manhattan, Carmel is sort of an older sister, mother, and shrink rolled into one. Boisterous and bubbly, with tight curls framing her face, she knows firsthand what the students are going through. She has lost 170 pounds in her own life, and worked at weight-loss camps for over a decade.

As a teenager, Carmel would have killed to go to a school like this. In fact, she designed one as a business model for a class at Cornell, from which she graduated in 1999. She knows how important it is for overweight kids to have a place where they feel secure, and an adult who really listens to them.

"They're victims of a culture assaulting them with mixed messages," she says. "With the conflicting messages of society, it's near impossible for anyone to lose weight. They don't really know what to do with Atkins, the Zone, or not eating fat or not eating late at night. If you're not going to give kids the kind of education they need, then it's a hopeless venture, which is why this school is the greatest place ever. We tell them what the fat is doing to them. I say in a very adolescent friendly manner, 'When you give your body fat it has a big huge party,' and it's like, 'Yes! I'm going to have a party and I'm going to grow big.' So, I think there's some reasoning that goes on when they see, 'Wow, that's 85 grams of fat and that's not something my body can really do and I don't know that it's worth it.'"

One night in mid-September, the kids gather in a common area separating the girls' wing from the boys'. They are discussing the Reedley Red, White and Blue parade, which is taking place the following Saturday. The students are encouraged to participate in it:

"We're part of the community now," says Craig. None of the kids are especially excited about it—Reedley, population 40,000, is not exactly a booming metropolis. (It's not even the raisin capital of the world anymore—that honor now goes to the neighboring town of Selma.)

"How about renting a big fat inflatable man, and his arm goes like this . . . ?" asks Terry Henry, gesturing like a cook flipping burgers on a grill. Terry arrived at AOS from Dallas weighing 550—the heaviest student so far. "What if we hand out Mardi Gras beads with AOS on them?"

Daniel Burger shakes his head. "What about we hold a banner that says, 'Losing weight, feeling great?'"

"Why are we handing stuff out?" a girl asks. "They're just going to make fun of us, the fat kids."

Suddenly the room grows quiet. No one has considered this before, or if they have, they haven't admitted it aloud. Being made fun of is something they're familiar with, and not something they want to deal with here.

Craig speaks up. "We're not going to force you to walk in the parade. I see your point. But it's a community and we're part of it. I'd just ask you to help us prepare, okay?"

The following week, they all marched in the parade. No one made fun of them.

» «

Five thousand, five hundred dollars a month is a lot of money to a lot of people, and AOS doesn't yet offer scholarships. Full insurance coverage is only available for Aspen's residential treatment centers, which are more like hospitals. But the therapy provided in their programs, including at AOS and Wellspring Camps, is reimbursable. Licensed therapists bill for hours spent with students or campers, and families are reimbursed about a quarter of the cost. (In October 2004, the Children's Aid Society of New York successfully won a court order requiring the State to pay the tuition for a

550-pound, fifteen-year-old boy who was literally eating himself to death, but that was an anomaly.)

Those who don't have any other options, find them. Like Stacey Fay, whose seventeen-year-old daughter, Jessica, arrived at AOS a few weeks after the first semester began. Jessica began gaining weight in the sixth grade, when she was diagnosed with paranoid schizophrenia and doctors plied her with pills. Eventually they got the mental illness under control, but the weight never disappeared, and it traumatized her. "The mental illness is nothing compared to the extra pounds," Fay recalls, glancing over at her daughter, who is about five foot four and 250 pounds. "She'd do her best to absolutely suck right into the walls because she doesn't want to be noticed. Kids walk by her and say, 'God, you're fat.' On one of her last days in school, four boys blocked the hall with about a foot between each one of them and said, 'Try to get through here, fatty.' I can tell her until I'm blue in the face, 'You're a wonderful person no matter how much you weigh, it's who you are on the inside that matters,' but it takes me days to undo what one boy says to her. If she could win this weight battle, I don't think there's anything in her mind she couldn't do."

One morning in early September, Jessica stayed home from school and saw a brief segment on *Good Morning America* about AOS. She immediately phoned her mom.

A single mother of two (her son does not have a weight problem), Fay, forty-two, works as a lab technician at the Mayo Clinic in Menomonie, Wisconsin, and she could ill afford the price of the school. But she knew how important this was to her daughter. It was a matter of life and death, so she took out a $70,000 student loan—the value of her house—to cover the costs.

"Jessica tried to commit suicide a few times," Fay recalls quietly. "If she ever succeeds I could accept it if I knew I tried everything for her. But I had to try everything. I thought, 'Well, if I could have my daughter, what's $70,000?' This is our last hope."

» «

Thanksgiving 2004 was the first time Kevin Marema went out into the real world since arriving at AOS two months earlier. He admits he was "really nervous" about going home. He worried about sticking to the food and exercise plan, even though the school held a mock Thanksgiving dinner, which the kids prepared themselves. The school also e-mailed parents a list of holiday Do's and Don'ts ("Stay positive and encourage your child"; "Promote activities in every way you can"; "Don't nag!") to eliminate any potential conflicts.

On his first night home, Kevin, his mother, and his older sister, Katie, went to an old friend's house for dinner. The friend had cooked a barbecue chicken and Kevin panicked; he didn't know how to monitor it. "I was a little upset, because I felt like I just need to eat it plain," he explains. He ultimately opted for salad instead of chicken, but the experience unnerved him.

"He does tend to be compulsive in many areas of his life when he's striving to reach goals," his mother says. "He has his act together enough that if they were not such good friends and he did not feel comfortable with them, he would not have said anything."

After that meal, he calmed down. In restaurants, he would look things up in his calorie book and would make the best choices possible. He even brought a set of measuring cups to T.G.I. Friday's.

His mother is thrilled by his diligence. "I believe it takes constant vigilance on the part of the parent to oversee whatever program might work for the child," she says. "A month at camp, a weekly visit to the nutritionist, a weekly to a therapist is not enough unless the parent is totally focused on the child with little or no other obligations in life. As you can well imagine, this is not the American Lifestyle of the day. I believe that the lifestyle change has to be reinforced constantly until the child gets it and makes it his own."

Kevin's father is a little more concerned. "I know fanaticism is probably necessary in the beginning, but he's got to learn not to force his behavior on the people around him," he says. "You can't walk into school and read the officials the riot act about what they can and can't serve in the food line, unless you want to be an activist. It's not like giving up alcohol; you can't abstain from food. You've got to learn to manage it."

On Thanksgiving Eve, Kevin enters the dining room wearing a black Mickey Mouse shirt and khaki shorts, carrying his journal and calorie book. He places them on the right side of his plate. There are just eight people here: his grandmother and her fiancé, an aunt and uncle and cousin, his mother and sister. His father is at an industry conference in Rio. Earlier in the week Kevin and his mother had flipped through the recipes the school had sent home. Rita cooked turkey, low-fat stuffing, low-fat gravy, a sweet potato, and vegetables. Kevin was in charge of the low-fat applesauce, made with apples and dietetic brown sugar.

He sits at one end of the table across from his mom, near the low fat food. The regular stuff, the "evil stuff" as his relatives jokingly call it, is at the other end. Kevin doesn't seem embarrassed or even worried about being judged. He knows what he needs to do, and he is doing it.

"What's school like?" Katie asks. Katie is surfer blonde and thin. (She is also adopted, which could explain the discrepancy in her weight.) "Do you all hang out together? Do you get sick of each other?"

"No," he says. "Everybody's really cool."

"Cool."

After dinner, Kevin clears the table, and then brings out the dessert plates and coffee cups. There is low-fat pumpkin pie (an AOS recipe) and an "evil" apple pie. Kevin cuts himself a slice of the pumpkin—"not so good"—and opts for some apple. Over the course of the night, he picks at the pie, popping gooey slices of apples inside his mouth. "That's the bad thing," his grandmother says, not unkindly.

Kevin shrugs. "I'll self-monitor what I eat," he says. An AOS victory: He was baited, he didn't bite. Success!

The Saturday after Thanksgiving he went with a family friend to Disney World. Yes, the unlimited food was a little overwhelming, but he found a place that served garden burgers and salads, and he walked 22,000 steps. By the time he returns to AOS two days later, he has lost three more pounds, for a total of thirty-three.

» «

Ryan Craig is pleased with the way things are going at the Academy of the Sierras. Thirty more kids have signed on for the second semester beginning in January, and the first group is doing remarkably well. About five kids stayed at school for Thanksgiving; of those who went home, only one binged. The kids self-monitored and followed the diet beautifully, although they didn't exercise nearly as much as he'd have hoped. So he and his staff developed a much more structured activity plan for each student, which the staff hoped the kids would follow over the Christmas break.

"We did quite a bit of parent education," says Craig. "We took about thirty minutes with each family to discuss it, and each student was given an individualized activity program which they committed to for the break." They also had a mock Christmas Dinner, preparing students to reenter an uncontrolled food environment. Of the eleven returning students, eight lost weight over the break.

Most of the kids—Kevin included—said they were eager to return to school, and several said they wished they hadn't even gone home. This surprised Craig. "I didn't think they'd want to get back to the grind," he says.

In Craig's ideal world, public schools across the country will adopt the AOS model: having kids self-monitor five minutes each morning and five minutes after school, and offering them in-depth nutrition and exercise classes. "Of course, we're not controlling the environment, but if we can get the school's support and begin to operationalize their thinking in that direction, we could help hundreds of thousands of kids each year."

Only time will tell what will happen once the first group leaves the Academy of the Sierras for good. Some will slip; others will maintain. Still others may end up getting surgery. A month before students are to return home for good, families will have to attend a two-day workshop, like the one offered by Camp Wellspring. The aftercare program lasts six months.

Kevin Marema thinks he'll do just fine once his time at AOS ends. Since September his clothes have gotten too big, and the features of his face are no longer submerged in flesh. He says he can't see the difference, though he feels it. He doesn't tire as quickly, he no longer huffs when he walks, and his joints don't ache. When he sees a photograph of himself from the summer, he murmurs, "God, look how fat I am." After all, "If I break 200, I get a trip to Disney Tokyo," he says, eyes shining.

» «

Ryan Craig is one of the few people I've encountered in the weight-loss world who impresses me. Sure, he's trying to make a profit, but his heart is in the right place. If he really wanted to make the big bucks he could have stayed in investment banking. But instead he's trying to build the best, most successful weight-loss program. I've seen him interact with his students, and believe he genuinely cares about and wants what's best for them.

My concern, though, is the same one I have for every controlled environment designed to curtail behavior. Granted, AOS—and to some extent the Wellspring Camps—are different from the other fat camps in that they offer a clinical model. Not only do students lose weight, they also learn something. And, of course, they get therapy.

But while Kevin and most of his school chums may have done beautifully during Thanksgiving and Christmas vacation, these were only short-term breaks. I worry what will happen to the kids when they go home for good, if they will be able to take their knowledge and implement it—and if so, for how long . . . ?

"Self-monitoring shows that people are watching their food intake and being vigilant about their calories," says Dr. Thomas Wadden, director of the weight and eating disorders program at the University of Pennsylvania School of Medicine. Wadden has conducted his own research on self-monitoring and found that the more food diaries one keeps, the greater the number of pounds one loses. Sure, people lie—people underestimate their food intake by about 40 to 50 percent—but "the fact that you're being vigilant means you'll probably eat fewer calories."

That said, "Even with self-monitoring, people are going to regain their weight," he says. "People tire of keeping food records. It works in the short term when you're getting support—when you lose weight it's exciting—the scale changes, your clothes fit better, your friends give you compliments. When you stop losing weight the band stops playing. You have to continue to keep records and to monitor and exercise regularly and you get no change—the scale stays constant. It's not very exciting, just as someone would never get excited if they worked and never got a raise.

"The biggest doubt I have with the school's method is will the behavior these kids have learned generalize when they go home? If you can create a nontoxic environment you'll lose weight. It's safe in schools and camps, but when you come out you're faced with all the pressures that cause you to gain weight. They have the tools, but which is stronger, their training, skills, and education, or a multibillion-dollar market that says eat this and play these video games? In the long term, it seems the environment wins."

He's painting a bleak picture, and I can't help hoping that maybe Ryan Craig and his school will slap the statistics in the face. Maybe the students at AOS will be the exceptions that disprove the rule. Maybe they'll self-monitor themselves into size 8s and never hear another word about being fat.

One can only hope.

2

behavior modification
and its discontents

a boarding school for overweight kids is a great idea. But say you don't have thousands of dollars at your disposal. Say you can barely afford to clothe your kids, let alone send them off for $5,500 a month. Maybe you work two jobs and have difficulty paying rent. Weight loss might be the least of your worries. Nutrition? Healthy eating? Please! Who can afford fresh fish? Who has time to cook?

Unfortunately, sometimes health issues kick in, and it's no longer okay (if it ever really was) for your child to carry around extra weight. Somehow, amid all the trials of daily life, you have to find a way to help your kid lose weight—without pawning your jewelry or mortgaging your house.

Lots of hospitals have in- and outpatient weight-loss programs, and for the most part they're all structured fairly similarly. Kids meet with doctors, endocrinologists, nutritionists—either by themselves or with their parents—and also participate in some kind of supervised physical activity. I spent some time at the Fit Matters Weight Control program at La Rabida Hospital in Chicago, run by one Daniel Kirschenbaum—who also works with the Academy of the Sierras.

The free program targets overweight lower income and minority families, and takes a cognitive-behavioral approach to weight loss, focusing not only on the behaviors of eating and exercise but also the thoughts and feelings that go into our behaviors. The goal is to change those thoughts "so we're more healthfully motivated," says Dr. Julie Germann, the program coordinator. There is a thirty-dollar initial fee to cover books and materials, including a pedometer. The family is required to have some type of insurance that will cover the medical costs of the program: seeing the pediatric endocrinologist, labwork, the physical therapist for the exercise group. Most families have Medicaid, which pays a tiny amount for the program. Private insurance typically doesn't pay for weight-loss programs; the families with private insurance only pay twenty dollars per group.

The National Institutes of Health report that 80 percent of African-American women and nearly 61 percent of men are overweight or obese, and 46 percent of African-American teens are overweight and 27 percent obese. (Anorexia, on the other hand, is rare among black women in the U.S., reports the July 2003 issue of the *American Journal of Psychiatry*.)

So far, about 250 families have gone through the La Rabida program, with the average group lasting about three to six months. But it's a tough diet to follow: only 1,200 calories and 20 grams of fat a day, just like the Academy of the Sierras. The goal is for each patient to walk 10,000 steps a day—between four and five miles—and lose 10 percent of his or her body weight. Besides the obvious health benefits, the program offers financial rewards. Each kid has a chance to earn two dollars in group: one dollar for writing in their journals every day "self-monitoring" and meeting their step and fat gram goals, and another for totaling their fat grams every day, even when they are consuming more than the recommended daily allowance. (I see their point, but I'm not sure a dollar is enough of an incentive.) When they've self-monitored and accumulated 1,000,000 steps, they're given gift certificates for athletic shoes (their steps are tracked weekly and posted on a little chart). "We also try to teach the parents about rewarding appropriate behavior, like allowing TV time after the journaling and exercise are done," says Germann.

On this brisk day in October, five African-American women sit around a table in a warm, airy room at the hospital. A scale stands against one side of the room; a blackboard with kids' names and goal weights leans against the back wall. Germann is discussing contracts the mothers have set up with their kids, a reward system designed to inspire (or bribe) the kids to lose weight.

"Last week we talked about how to negotiate an individual reward between parents and kids as a motivator to lose weight," says Germann. "How do you all negotiate the reward system?"

The women take turns sharing. "Rehanna did well with exercise and calories counseling, but we need to make sure our meals are balanced," says Millie.

"But how did you negotiate the individual reward?" Germann asks.

"We decided to have a day where she could have what she wants," says Helen, a thin, pretty woman whose hair is slicked off her face in a tight ponytail. "But it's a watched day. She doesn't really go over, so it gives her structure. I still monitor her."

Pam says her leveling agent is the cell phone. "If you lose weight, you get the phone. If not, no."

Kyle Yates's mom, Karen, wears an orange fleece jacket, jeans, and sneakers. She is soft and well-spoken. Kyle has been at La Rabida for six months, but only recently has he embraced the program. "Now, he's very aware of what he's eating," she says. "His sister lost forty pounds, and he's become conscious of being overweight and unhealthy. He loves girls. The other day he met a girl who gave him her phone number. It turns out it was a rejection line—when you called it the voice on the machine said, 'If you're receiving this you are either too fat, too ugly, or too short and you need to be laughed at.' He was upset about the girl, but didn't cry."

"I'm excited about losing the weight *I'm* losing," says Carol, another mother. "I'm working out with a personal trainer. I've already changed Sonya's habits. I tried to limit sweets because she'll sneak to buy things—I know she's not motivated in this. But I know she's twelve years old and that's going to change. It's been a very long haul."

"What was her reward?" Germann asks.

"I tried to negotiate with buying new clothes and shoes if she'd exercise and eat what I feed her. But she won't exercise; I've got to get her signed up at a gym. So, negotiating didn't help at all. It didn't get her to do what she needs to do."

It didn't help me either, I want to say. Neither a trip to Florida nor a new wardrobe nor the promise of boys galore—nothing. You can't bribe someone to lose weight or stop smoking or do anything unless they want to do it. Maybe it works at first—maybe—but long-term studies of work incentives, behavior management programs for children, and weight-loss and smoking-cessation plans have all found that performance and quality of work declines over time because people are thinking only about the incentive or reward, instead of the value of what they're actually doing.

Teresa knows about this. "I've had a terrible month just existing," she says. "My workload has been so heavy, so I've been negligent in trying to monitor Jordan. But we still go grocery shopping together, she reads the labels and I'm encouraged. She wants fat free; she reads the papers and looks for bargains. We joined a health club where parents can go and the child costs ten dollars extra. She likes it and it forces *me* to go. The other day I wanted to sleep in and she says, 'We gotta go to the health club!' We spent an hour and a half there." (It's amazing that Teresa even found a place where her daughter can work out, as most health clubs, probably for insurance reasons, don't let in kids under age fourteen.)

A heavy woman in a black suede coat with long silver nails says this about her daughter, Jill Ann, who spent four weeks as an inpatient at La Rabida. "Everything she ate, she had to exercise it off. Since she's left the hospital she's lost twelve pounds; she's down a full dress size. Everyone who sees her says, 'Jill Ann, you're getting so skinny!' The expression on her face is wonderful."

The mothers leave and then the kids, who have been lounging in the waiting room, saunter in: four girls and one boy. Let it be said, they are big, so big they have difficulty walking up stairs, down hallways, fitting in desks. But they know it. That, after all, is why they are here.

First matter of business: weigh-in.

This is not greeted with whoops and hollers. Weigh-in is serious stuff, the fat person's polygraph test. The kids just sit there until Kyle Yates, twelve, the lone boy in the group, volunteers. He steps up to the scale in a red shirt and blue sweat pants that are three sizes too big; he is up 0.2 pounds and he is perplexed. How can this have happened? He's been good all week. Rehanna, who is small on top but has a large rear end, is down 2.2 pounds. Jill is down half a pound; Sonya is down 2.2. Jordan, the biggest girl, is up 3.2.

Germann is pleased. Kids often gain weight (a girl in another group has gained seventy-five pounds since she began the program, but since Germann sees her "potential," she didn't kick her out) and so she's happy when the numbers go the other way. I appreciate Germann's optimism, but it seems counterproductive—not to mention demoralizing—to allow a kid who gains weight to stay in the program.

Next, she talks about journaling. Have they been keeping an activity log? Have they been writing down what they've eaten, how much they've exercised, how many grams of fat they've consumed?

The kids crack gum and squirm. Clearly, they would rather be anywhere but here. Only Rehanna has completed her log. Germann hands her two crisp dollar bills.

Then they move on to other pressing points, namely, The Olive Garden Matter.

A few weeks earlier, one of the mothers came up with the idea that maybe a group reward would help inspire weight loss. This thought had been bandied about. Parents, it seemed, were more excited about this than the kids. And it was difficult to execute. First they had to settle on a place, which was a lot harder than it sounded. Not all of the kids liked Olive Garden (one kid blithely suggested Chuck E. Cheese, which was quickly vetoed), and perhaps more important, the kids' ages varied. The thought of sharing a meal with someone four years younger wasn't particularly enticing.

And there was the problem of semantics. The way Germann understood the plan, everyone had to have lost five pounds three weeks after the initial conversation took place. From the kid's perspective, though, anyone who lost five pounds in *total* would be allowed to go to the Olive Garden.

The topic is now up for discussion. "The goal was to lose five pounds in three weeks," she said. "Kyle did—6.8. Jordan lost 5 but gained some back. Jill lost 4.5 pounds. Sonya lost 3 and gained back 2. So, was it 5 pounds in general or 5 pounds by today? Does the whole group get to go or just the people who meet the goal?"

Kyle raises his hand. In his opinion, majority should rule; whoever wants to go should go. "People who met their goals should be rewarded," he says.

"You did work hard these past two weeks," she says to him. "So, congrats on doing the work. What helped you be successful?"

"My motivation is girls," says Kyle with a broad grin. He's affable and the most vocal of the lot, with a sweet, open face. "You gotta look nice for the girls. I believe losing weight for girls is good, but it's better to lose weight for you."

What else?

Kyle grins broadly. "Maybe getting teased. When you get teased at school you get tired of it. I'm gonna lose enough weight so they stop teasing me. And if they keep doing it, they're just jealous."

Back to the Olive Garden. Germann wants to know if they're worried about eating there, if the thought of going to a restaurant—and not pigging out—is daunting.

"I'm not worried," says Kyle. "You get soup and salad and bread sticks. I'll bring my own dressing, fat-free ranch." He oozes confidence.

Rehanna flips through *The Doctor's Pocket Calorie, Fat, and Carbohydrate Counter,* one of three books the kids are given. (They also get a journal to list food, calories, and fat grams, as well as the number of steps taken and exercise completed, and *The Nine Truths about Weight Loss,* by Daniel Kirschenbaum, but at 237 pages it seems unlikely that anyone actually reads it.)

She looks up the calorie count for the Olive Garden. Minestrone soup has 100 calories; a bread stick has 140 calories, with one gram of fat. Not bad at all. But what to do?

The mothers are called back in.

Germann is polite but firm. "They're right—there was effort, but I didn't expect them to lose five and gain seven," she says.

"I think if we're doing it collectively everyone should go, regardless if they met their goals," says one mother.

Another says: "I think it should be left up to the kids. If they wanna go, I'm all for it."

They decide to vote by secret ballot. Final verdict: Everyone who wants to will go.

After group, the moms and the kids trudge down the hall for a nutrition lecture run by the terminally peppy dietitian intern Tina Musselman, twenty-three, who I later learn weighed 220 pounds as a kid. She is around 170 now, but she's tall: five foot ten. The irony of her last name—muscle-man—has not escaped her, or me.

I had actually noticed her downstairs by the vending machines earlier in the day, when I was waiting for group to start. She was heating food in the microwave while I was trying to get change. The experience was slightly maddening. There was not one healthy snack at the hospital, in either the vending machines or the cafeteria—no apples or bananas or even PowerBars, although there were plenty of Dove bars, Klondikes, chicken wings, Cheetos, Fritos, and Famous Amos cookies. I found this significant. How are doctors supposed to inspire their charges to be healthy when the hospital— which runs wellness programs for employees (many of whom are quite overweight)—serves highly caloric food? Who are they kidding? I ended up with a pepperoni stuffed Hot Pocket and a diet Mountain Dew, which has more caffeine than a Diet Coke.

Germann understands my annoyance. She usually brings her own food from home. Alas, "It's not economically feasible for the hospital to serve healthy food," she says. An apple isn't economically feasible? (She explains that fast food is very common in both public and private hospitals across the country for financial reasons—

McDonald's, for example, gives money to charities that benefit hospitals, like the Ronald McDonald House program, and has outlets in many hospitals across the country. Welcome to America, land of the paradox.)

Tonight's topic: the link between calcium and weight loss.

"Where can you get dairy?" Musselman asks.

The group shouts out answers: "Butter!" "Cheese!" "Ice Cream!"

Yes, yes, and yes—except Musselman was looking for, uh, healthier answers. She adds: Broccoli. Kale. Raw spinach. Yogurt. Milk (preferably low fat). Calcium-fortified orange juice. Canned sardines (with bones).

Musselman cites a study that found that patients who eat three to four servings of dairy while cutting calories can lose twice the weight of those who just decreased calories.

She tells the families to stay away from soda (it's the Midwest, so she calls it pop), since it depletes calcium. So do caffeine and alcohol. "If you use a dairy supplement, space it an hour and a half after you eat for absorption," she says.

Then she brings out a range of low-fat calcium-rich food—Jell-O, yogurt, low-fat cheese, fat-free pudding, cottage cheese, canned fish with bones—for everyone to taste. Everyone is happy to be eating, and who would have thought fat-free pudding could taste so good and be so good for you?

All the same, this information is a lot to digest. It feels like so much work to eat right. And if I feel that way, they must, too.

Musselman is well aware of this. "Knowledge is great, but if you don't do anything with it, it doesn't do any good," she says.

» «

The next day Germann and I meet in her office. She eats a chicken salad, which she brought from home. I have a turkey on whole wheat sandwich, no mayo, that I got in the hospital cafeteria—the healthiest thing there—a bottle of water and a Diet Coke. In my bag I have a Reese's peanut butter cup and a Twix, which I chow down when she leaves. All this food talk makes me hungry.

I like Julie right away. "We have the kids journal at night. It helps with the weight loss. It's constant mindfulness." (I decide not to comment on the Dalai Lama approach.)

But only if they tell the truth.

Which brings me to my next point. Nutritionists and diet experts have long advised dieters to write down what they've eaten, and I've certainly done my share of journaling. On paper, I was the model dieter, a pillar of caloric control. But in real life? Moo. I was never honest. I didn't want to write down all that I ate. I knew I had overeaten, so why did I need to put it on paper? Frankly, it was no one's business.

Germann knows this is a problem. "Sometimes you want to say to them, 'How do you walk so much and eat nothing and yet gain weight?' A lot of kids resist it—it's a pain to do, it's tedious, you have to look up stuff in a calorie book and wear the pedometer—although it takes all of five or ten minutes a day. But the kids who want to dig down and see what they can do to be healthier and find out how habits impact them do it. If they're not ready to do journaling in some way, they're not going to be successful—unless it's a younger kid and the parent gets the information and provides it in the home." Hmm. I wonder about that.

Germann is thirty-one and slim, with shoulder-length dark blonde hair and big eyes. She is rather chic, dressed in jeans and a funky T-shirt. She has a Ph.D. in clinical psychology, and did her postdoctorate in pediatric psychology. Her dissertation was on juvenile delinquency—that is, the connection between abuse and delinquency. She seems very dedicated and very good with her charges, although I wonder if perhaps she's too sweet and not hard enough on them. The hospital is very clean and bright, with cheery painted walls and floors. It's very unclinical—cozy, even—and everyone is so relentlessly friendly.

Germann got into the fat trade by accident, partly through her interest in delinquent kids and partly because of her own heartache. Her mother died nine years ago of congestive heart failure.

"My mother was overweight as long as I remember," she says. "I thought, there are enough things out there that can kill you, why not do everything you can to be healthy?" Germann didn't want to be "impaired" in any way, so she adopted a healthy lifestyle herself and dropped twenty pounds. Her father and brother have high blood pressure and cholesterol but neither one has done anything to change it.

"What's that about?" I ask. "What makes one person say, 'There are enough things that will kill me so I'm gonna be healthy' and another say, 'You never know when you're gonna die so bring on the donuts!' Why are there some glass-half-empty people and other half-full?"

Germann shrugs and smiles ruefully. If she knew that, she'd be God.

But one thing is clear: It takes a lot of work to change a behavior, especially for those of low socioeconomic status (SES). Most live with single mothers who are usually holding down one or two jobs and struggling to keep it all together. This creates a great challenge—and a lot of frustration—for everyone involved.

"The low SES has so many stresses: balancing a budget, keeping the gas and electricity on, keeping their kids safe," says Germann. Their lifestyle is so much more chaotic than the wealthier families on the North side of the city, where she also has an office. "They have poor health and poor life organization. They can't focus on weight issues because they're trying too hard to keep house. North families have a lot less chaos—they have insurance, they don't live paycheck-to-paycheck, they have transportation. Those kids will be successful because they have more resources and underlying advantages."

Indeed, federal statistics indicate that the higher the poverty level, the higher the rate of obesity, especially among minorities. Around 16 percent of whites who earn $50,000 are obese, but that figure climbs to nearly 23 percent among whites who only earn $15,000. Twenty-two percent of blacks who earn $50,000 are obese, compared with 34 percent for those in the $15,000 bracket.

A 1999 A. C. Nielsen Home Scan survey monitoring consumer

patterns among 55,000 households revealed that blacks dispropor-
tionately tended towards frozen and canned goods, pork products
and starches. While Latinos were more likely to purchase vegetables, they also bought fatty foods, like lard and refried beans.

A 2001 study from the University of Chicago Children's Hospital
found that blacks watch an average of seventy-five hours of TV a
week, compared to fifty-two hours in white households. Black kids
eat 62 percent of their meals in front of the TV, compared with 43
percent of Hispanic kids, 32 percent of white kids, and 21 percent of
Asian-American kids. Dr. Anjali Jain, the lead author, found that
there are more overweight characters (27 percent, compared with 2
percent on general prime-time shows), more food and drink commercials (4.178 per half hour versus 2.89, with 30 percent featuring
food and 13 percent featuring soda), and more actual food items (67
percent to 53 percent) on prime-time TV shows geared toward a
black audience than a white one.

"Wealthier parents bug kids differently," adds Daniel Kirschenbaum, who also has an office on Chicago's North Shore and is a professor of psychiatry and behavioral sciences at Northwestern
University Medical School. A small, earnest man with a neatly
trimmed beard and tiny gray pony tail, Kirschenbaum doesn't quite
look the part of obesity expert. If you didn't know he was a doctor,
you might think he was a game-show host. "When we ask parents
to get involved—it's required for participation—we ask at least one
parent to self-monitor, so they're modeling and learning with the
kid. They sign a contract before agreeing to do it. But we can't
maintain or enforce it because so few parents among the lower income people do it. At La Rabida maybe 25 percent of the parents
will do any monitoring at all. At my office downtown, we work with
wealthier kids and adults. They monitor 100 percent. I can't remember a parent who won't do it. There's more detachment in the
lower income family." (Or, I might suggest, more single parents trying to keep their heads above water.)

There's also a higher acceptable weight limit in the black community. In January, the Sinai Health Institute at Mt. Sinai Hospital,

in Chicago, found that 74 percent of youngsters aged six to twelve in the South Side of the city were considered overweight or obese, compared to 22 percent in middle-class and predominantly white areas. "With our population here at La Rabida there's nagging from parents, but usually the parents have weight problems, and some of the siblings do, too," says Germann. "There's a hereditary component. A lot of these kids turn to food for celebration—it's comfort, it's their automatic thing to do. Plus, there are so many social activities with food. We encourage them to pack lunches when they can, but it's expensive."

Kirschenbaum believes that self-control can be taught just like any other skill. "It's like learning to ride a bike," he says. "It's a process in behavioral terms, keeping track of target behaviors and systematically evaluating these behaviors, goal-setting and monitoring, evaluation, self-awareness."

Okay. But what if a kid doesn't want to follow a plan of action? Then what?

"First you work with the parents, if they're at least willing to participate," Kirschenbaum says. "Once they're shown the yellow brick road you see if they're gonna follow it. If they work at it for a while and the environment doesn't support it very well and they get depressed or don't care about size—they think size is good, especially with boys—we say, 'At least you know the right way to do this.' If at some point you want to do this, you have the information."

Germann agrees. A successful weight loss comes when "the whole family makes the change and they live it at home," she says. "A lot of the kids have reasons to lose weight: They want to shop, they want to attract the opposite sex, or play sports. But they don't live that. That's why it's so important for parents to instill it in them. The problem is, how do you change a house? We encourage them to make gradual changes, one thing at a time. The number one reason parents say they want their kid to lose weight is health. But some parents come in and don't know how to set limits and structures—basic parenting skills. I remember one kid who had three peanut butter sandwiches for dinner. He had no idea how unhealthy that is. For those kids it's difficult to make changes in this kind of program because there are so many other issues and no one is controlling them."

"Maybe the parents are just happy that their kids aren't smoking crack," I say. "In comparison, a candy bar isn't so bad."

"Yes, but these kids are heart attacks waiting to happen."

Indeed, most of the La Rabida kids have some kind of health issue, like sleep apnea, insulin resistance, high cholesterol, or all three. Some take meds. One girl was given a prescription for Meridia, but her insurance didn't cover it so she had to stop. Another took Xenical, but she still wasn't losing weight. "It's a fat blocker, so if she's doing what she's supposed to be doing—eating low-fat and low-cal foods—then there's no fat for her to block," Germann says. "So that makes sense."

"Then why was she on it?" I ask.

"They think it's a quick fix."

As for the dreaded scale, Germann thinks it's helpful to weigh yourself daily. "I do it, and for me it's just like the daily journaling, it keeps me mindful of my weight all the time," she says, admitting that she has been known to step on more than once a day. "If I don't weigh myself for a long time I don't know what's going on. It depends what the individual issues are, though—for people who are obsessed with their weight and underweight then that can be damaging because it's too much of a preoccupation. But when people are really significantly overweight or have the tendency to be that way—like I do—it's helpful to weigh yourself every day."

What's the biggest challenge with her patients?

"All of the moms have made positive changes—they really have come a long way," she says. "Some of them say sadly, 'This is my fault. We both used food for comfort. I should have nipped this years ago.' What gets frustrating is when you see families doing well but there are some areas where there's blatant disregard. I need to remember that they're not perfect. In general, we recommend that beef and pork are high fat and you want to avoid them. Juice, too, especially, for those kids with diabetes. Then they'll talk about a time when they barbecued ribs or whatever. The rationalization is that every once in a while isn't going to kill you, and it's not."

I'm curious about the Olive Garden. Why was food the reward? "Isn't the whole point to get away from using food as rewards?"

"Good question," she says, popping a piece of chicken into her mouth. "My first inclination was, 'Why are we rewarding with food?' But it gets at motivation. For a lot of kids just losing weight isn't enough—you need to figure out what's motivating them and it has to be immediate enough. For Sonya, for example, a weekly reward isn't good enough. Maybe it needs to be daily—like, you can't watch TV until you do your homework. That's the basis of behavior modification: positive reinforcement."

This has been as much of a learning experience for Germann as it has been for her patients. One week, for example, everyone gained weight, so she decided not to focus on weight loss and instead focused on exercise. They also negotiated a specific reward—that is, if they didn't accomplish their goals they lost privileges, like cell phone use or TV.

(I have to wonder: Is it positive reinforcement to remove a cell phone or TV that you then allow them to use only as a reward for performance? From a kid's point of view, to start a system now, when they're already undisciplined, might seem less a positive reinforcement than a punishment).

And wouldn't you know it—the next week everyone lost weight. "What we realized, as with the Olive Garden, is that a group reward doesn't motivate. It's hard to get a group consensus, and some kids don't care about being with the group. So individual motivation and rewards are more of the key."

And though it can be like continually bumping your head against the wall, she is hopeful.

"What keeps me going are the little changes you see the families make," she says. "Not just the numbers, but what else is changing. Going to the gym, finding a trainer, hearing the kids so excited about exercising. We plant a lot of seeds—it's a ton of information—but hopefully one or two of those will bloom somewhere along the way. Often when they make one or two changes and it gets rolling and it's so gratifying."

» «

The next day Kathy, a social worker, runs the show. As always, the session begins with weigh-in.

Albert is up half a pound. He doesn't understand how this can be, so he takes off his sweatshirt and heads back to the scale. Score! It's the same as last week.

Then there is AJ, fourteen, who is bigger than anyone I have seen in my life, even in all the fat-farm years. His right eye is bloody, as if a vessel has exploded inside it, and he is filled with rage. Every scale he weighs himself on says something different: He was 420 at one place, 383, and 333. Tonight he is 432, and he is pissed.

"I really don't care anymore," he says. "I busted my butt. I'm here every week for an hour."

"Why do you want to do this?" Kathy asks.

"So I can do things and so I don't get treated like I'm different," he says. "There's nothing left to do but get surgery."

He sounds like an old man, his breathing heavy, his inability to stand up without exerting enormous effort. "I don't look like I'm 400. I don't feel 400. This weight junk is confusing and giving me a headache."

Kathy placates him in that therapist speak I find so patronizing. "I understand your frustration," she says. To me, that's right up there with "I feel your pain" or "I hear how unhappy you are"— textbook shrink catchphrases designed to placate the patient. Have *you* ever been 400 pounds? I want to yell. She should say, "I'm sorry you have deal to with this. I wish you didn't have to live like this. You've got a bum deal. But let's try to change it."

"I got a blood-infested eye because kids at school thought they could talk about me and I wouldn't get mad. I'm not gonna take that. I should forget about this and just get surgery. Just get me the surgery."

» «

AJ would be an excellent candidate for La Rabida's inpatient program, which is for kids who absolutely cannot get it together on their own. For eight weeks patients—most of whom are battling sleep apnea, asthma, diabetes, cardiac problems, and high blood pressure—live in the hospital under intense medical supervision. In addition to daily exercise classes and psychology sessions, they meet with a physical therapist five hours a week, a dietitian two to three times per week, and continue to attend the weekly group meetings. (All inpatient participants must attend the weekly outpatient program for at least one month before they can be admitted for a lengthy stay. There's also a Chicago public school teacher on board so the kids can theoretically stay current with homework.) Patients are weighed twice a week, once with the dietitian at the beginning of each week and once during group. The goal is to lose 10 percent of their body weight in the time they are there, a goal just about all weight-loss programs prescribe.

A week costs $1,500, which is paid for by Public Aid (private insurance won't authorize it—they view it as a weight-loss program, which most insurance will not cover).

Postdischarge success depends on the level of family commitment. Those without it usually regain the weight (and more), but those with very involved families and a strong commitment continue to lose.

"The rationale is that if they're not able to be compliant here in a very structured environment, they're not ready to go out to the real world," says Germann. "It's a privilege the kids work hard for, so the home pass is an ideal motivator for a behavioral plan."

Unless, of course, you don't want to go home. And why would you, if your mother introduced you to people with this happy line: "This is my daughter Domnique. Ain't she big?"

Domnique Gregory tells me this with a laugh, but it's clearly a painful memory. How could it not be? Domnique is a bubbly and articulate seventeen-year-old who has been at La Rabida for seven weeks when I meet her. She couldn't wait to go into the hospital. Other than a minor case of sleep apnea, she's healthy, but she's five foot five and weighs 252 pounds and wants to lose one hundred pounds. She has lost twelve pounds in the hospital, not nearly as much as she expected or hoped, but it's better than nothing, and certainly better than gaining. And she has gone down two dress sizes, which is nice.

No one seems to know why she's not losing more. "I exercise all day, but my body will not let this fat go," she says. "The doctors don't know why. First, they say it's a plateau. Then, it's water weight. Then, I'm gaining muscle. I used to say I wanted to be a certain size by prom. Now I don't look at the numbers."

Domnique, who coils her braided hair tightly atop her head, is a senior in high school and hopes to study psychology in college, with a minor in drama. Her weight problem began when she was seven, when she, her brother, and mother moved from the city to the suburbs, and she sat around, watched TV, and "was a loner," she explains.

She would skip breakfast and stuff herself with chips and soda at lunch. Then she'd come home and hit the tube. For dinner her mom, Jordan, fifty-three, would make fried chicken with macaroni and cheese on the side, and give her Pepsi to drink. When her mom was out—she worked two jobs at one point—Domnique ate pizza and Hostess Twinkies and cupcakes that Jordan brought home from her job at a bulk-discount store. "I never wanted her to suffer for anything," says Jordan, who's a diabetic who has weathered colon and bladder surgeries, "but what I did was isolate her at home. My mistake."

Life in the suburbs was painful. "One girl would say, 'Your kneecaps are so big!'" Domnique recalls with a laugh. (I am wide-eyed. Amazing, some of the creativity behind fat barbs. Who looks at kneecaps?)

The family returned to the city three years later, when Domnique was entering the fifth grade. That's when her mom started making comments about her weight.

"I'm the biggest of all my cousins," Domnique says. "I'm the outsider in my family. My cousins have brown or red hair, long curly hair. I'm different. I didn't know my Dad—I have four brothers and we all have different dads—but my mom says I'm built like his sisters, with a big chest. No one in my family is big like me."

Her mom was a "looker" who would try to dress her daughter the way she dressed when *she* was young, in tight shirts and short skirts. In her mother's eyes, Domnique would be perfect if only she "got braces, let her hair grow longer, and lost weight."

"I tried to diet, but I didn't know what to do," Domnique says. "I'd just try not to eat. In the fifth grade I weighed 180—if I ate chips my family would say, 'What are you doing?' So I'd eat it right in their face."

She learned about La Rabida from her doctor. She joined the outpatient group, and then chose to go inhouse. She's not embarrassed; all of her friends know she's there. "The good friends I have are all pretty," she says. "Two of them are like sticks, and the third has the shape of a Coca-Cola bottle. One of them would say to the other, 'Oh, you're getting fat.' Well, I'd think, 'If she's fat, what does that make me?'"

"I have a friend who's bigger than me," she continues. "She says I sold out the big girls by coming here. I tell her I'm gonna work out with her. She's always depressed about how she looks."

Life is a little boring in the hospital: Wake up at 9 A.M. for breakfast. Go to school until 11:30. Have lunch at noon. At 1 P.M., see Julie, or go to physical therapy (where she jumps rope, bikes, lifts weights), or visit the nutritionist. Dinner is at 5 P.M., usually a chicken breast and corn. After, go to the playroom, watch TV, or use the computer. Repeat the next day, and the next.

Despite the monotony, Domnique is happy here. Why not? She gets a lot of respect—she's kind of like the floor mama. The younger kids adore her, and the nurses treat her like a friend. Really, it's been a blessing to be out of her house. "Sometimes I get bored, but I'm a loner anyway and kind of shy," she says. "The people are great. You get a lot of encouragement and advice—what you should get at home. But my mother's really controlling. She is so negative.

Everyone tells her I'm great, still a virgin, don't do anything bad, get straight As, go to church."

Although her mother bugs Domnique about her weight, she was a lousy role model. "She would have Pepsi, salad with regular dressing, fried chicken, and still tell me to lose weight," Domnique recalls. "She'd say, 'You know you're not supposed to eat that,' while she's eating cake and drinking Coke. I don't think she knows the concepts, and she's not fat.

"When your child feels it's the time to lose weight, encourage her," she continues. "Nobody wants to be singled out—like, only telling one child that she needs to lose weight but not telling the others. Everyone should eat healthy; it's not going to work if one kid's eating broccoli and everyone else is eating pizza. Then the kid will run out and eat. So make it a family thing."

Domnique feels like her weight is stopping her in life. "I always cared about my weight—I'm a big dreamer and wisher and I wish I wasn't like this," she admits. "But now I'm older and I know wishes aren't going to cut it. I'm waiting on college. I used to say, 'I'm going to lose weight for me and I'm going to show them.' I don't think you should be trying to get back at them, but that's how I feel.

"I love everything—I'm interested in kickboxing, writing a movie script, going to a garden, looking at flowers," she adds. "I want to run a marathon. I want to be an actress. It won't happen— you don't see people like me on TV. I used to take acting and modeling and talent classes at John Robert Powers. I was the biggest person in the place. They let me in, I paid, but it wasn't fun for me and I left. Now I just wanna feel good."

As for leaving—she has one week left in the hospital—she is conflicted. "I'm excited to see what I can do on my own. I already know my mom's gonna be difficult. I tell myself I'm not going to be in the house until it's time to go to sleep."

Germann thinks Domnique will continue to be successful; of all the kids in group, she's progressed the most, and she seems to be committed and motivated. And she didn't sneak food, or, like one kid, "bribe somebody to get food out of the vending machines, or, like another kid, have a pizza delivered to the front desk," Germann says. She has high hopes for Domnique.

» «

Germann, it turns out, is wrong.

When Domnique first left the hospital, twenty pounds lighter in total, she walked everyday and steered clear of her mother's fried chicken. She felt pretty good, her friends were supportive, and she was pumped.

She changed her diet to include oatmeal for breakfast, salads and low-fat sandwiches for lunch, and ate grapes and oranges as snacks. She joined a Bally Total Fitness health club, and really "tried to make the commitment on my own."

That lasted a few weeks. Then Life got in the way. For one thing, her brother is back on drugs. And it's crazy at home: She goes to sleep at 1 A.M. and gets up at 6. Part of it is trying to stay afloat at school. Though she had a teacher at La Rabida, the work was just busy work. "One teacher even gave me an F, for what I don't know," she says.

But she loved the hospital. It taught her what to eat and how to exercise. Unfortunately, some of the weight came back—"because I didn't have any money so I ate noodles and things like that; but then I'd exercise for an hour straight. It was only a pound or two."

She never went back to La Rabida, and never returned Germann's calls.

» «

So, what gives? Why are some people successful and others, not? To be sure, there is the amount of weight they need to lose—ten pounds is one thing, 110 is quite another. And there's the issue of how much effort goes into losing each pound, and how long it takes to do it.

Tina Musselman, the former intern at Fit Matters, thinks the diet is a large part of the problem there. "It's unrealistic," she says.

"When I was in high school I would never think of counting calories versus just eating healthy and being active. The program is a great concept, but the nutrition part could have used a little help. Twenty grams of fat a day is *low*; I can't imagine it. But I did like the psychological component and the multidisciplinary approach."

It's also easy to get discouraged. Even Julie Germann is exhausted by the whole process of losing and maintaining weight—and she's thin.

"For me personally, it's difficult that it's about lifestyle change, but also that it never ends," she says. "There's never a termination. It's always a struggle and there's no closure to it. Even if kids are successful and get down to their healthy weight, it just goes on and on and on."

» «

That's exactly what Kyle Yates thinks.

Now 235, he's lost fifteen pounds since starting Fit Matters in July 2003. He's also shot up, from five foot four to five foot eight, and he started riding his bike the four and a half miles to school. He's curbed his appetite—sort of. "Now I eat three or four chips and the bag will last me for the whole month. I have this little thing on the phone and on the fridge and in my wallet: It says, 'Lose weight, get more clothes.' I just think about all the new clothes I could get, and it helps me stay straight."

That, and, oh, yeah, Girls. "I like girls a lot. That's the top reason why I want to lose," he says with a laugh.

It's taken some time to get used to all this, though. "When I first came in the group I was the quiet one. But then I started opening up more. But it's so hard. You wanna eat all the fattening chips like you used to and the greasy hamburger, but you gotta step away from it." In the wintertime there's nothing for him to do. He comes home from school, turns on the TV, and does his homework. His mom, a security guard in a grammar school, doesn't get in until after six. "That was always a big opportunity for me to get junk food," he says.

Since he and his mom started the program, she has changed the entire food inventory in the house. She keeps fruit around, bakes instead of fries, and serves vegetables every night.

Kyle's not sure how he got fat. He was very energetic as a kid—he used to swim, and even won first place in nationals. But then he started wheezing and his doctor gave him an asthma pump. "There's really steroids in the pump and that's why I gained weight. You get muscles from steroids," says Kyle. "I was eating a lot and getting fatter. It's kinda hard to do things when you've got that much weight."

He's been in private school since December of 2002. He had to go—the kids kept teasing him at the public school. "I kept getting jumped on in the hallway for being fat," he says matter-of-factly. "In swimming class they called me Shamu, and they peed on my clothes. A teacher smelled my clothes and he said, 'It's not pee.' The principal said it wasn't either. I told my mama and she said, 'You're outta there.'"

He likes private school because "they help me. We have off-campus lunch and I would go out and buy snacks and stuff, and one time I had a bag of Flaming Hots and the kids snatched the bag and said, 'We're trying to help you even though we talk about you.'" With friends like that . . .

Fit Matters helps him, he says. If he wasn't in the program he'd probably slack off. "It's good to know that there are other people in the group who have problems," he says. In his ideal world, he'd like to spend the summer at fat camp. But he can't afford it.

Still, he is determined to lose weight. "I'm gonna keep on going until I get down to 160."

Kyle spent two years with Fit Matters, until he left it behind for the football team. Football helped stop the teasing. "People don't mess with me because they know I have protection," he says, noting that he lost more weight on the football team than at the hospital program. Now a high-school freshman, he says he's getting a lot more attention from the girls. He didn't get down to his goal weight of 160; 235 was the best he could do. That's ok. "I'm happy with that," he says.

» «

Researchers seriously began studying weight loss in the 1950s, and behavior modification became the most widely used method for long-term success. The goal is to change eating habits, and make new ones, by creating new behavior patterns. Most programs recommend developing new habits like reading a newspaper instead of eating, eating before going shopping, and keeping a food diary.

The behavior modification movement stems from a 1967 University of Michigan study, "Behavioral Control of Overeating," which analyzed self-control as it applied to weight loss. The author, Richard B. Stuart, studied eight overweight women who had recurrent meetings with a therapist and kept a food log and mood journal. They lost twenty-five to forty-seven pounds a year.

Fit Matters is one of a handful of in- and outpatient hospital programs in the country that use a mixture of behavior modification, nutrition and exercise classes, and parental involvement.

In the 1950s, B. F. Skinner, generally considered the father of behavior-modification sciences, trained rats and children to reproduce behavior patterns through a system of punishment and reward. He eventually recanted some of his earlier conclusions. He reached the understanding that what holds for rats may not apply to humans, who are driven by deeper levels of incitement. If there is a loss of interest in the reward, people become less motivated to do the task, or they just endure it to reap the benefit. Instead of trying to do the best job, they take shortcuts. Ideally, they would be doing something to please themselves and not a parent or doctor.

But how do you inspire kids to do something to please themselves and not a parent or doctor? Ten-year-old Clara Lay and her mom, Alicia, a registered nurse, live in Independence, Ohio. They joined Healthworks!, part of the Heart Center at Cincinnati Children's Hospital Medical Center, in August 2003. The program caters to overweight children ages five to ten and adolescents eleven to nineteen. By December 2004, Clara had lost twenty-five pounds — not an insignificant amount for a five-foot, 123-pound kid.

Like Fit Matters, Healthworks! emphasizes diet modification, physical activity, behavior therapy, parental involvement, and group exercise sessions offered by age group. While the kids work out, the adult family members meet with dietitian Shelly Kirk at least once a month to learn about nutrition, physical activity, and weight management. Like Fit Matters, it's also goal-oriented. The child comes up with a weekly goal and gets a reward of his choice for meeting it.

Clara's problem wasn't one of mere aesthetics, though (after all, she wasn't *that* big). Her mother was genuinely worried about her health. Over time a dark ring had formed around her neck, knuckles, and knees. "It looked like she needed to wash her neck really bad," Alicia says. "We were concerned she had a cortisol problem."

So they took her to an endocrinologist, who proclaimed her insulin resistant. Plus, "She was heavy and lethargic and not very involved and hung out in her bedroom all the time," her mother says. And she was teased. One time her mother took her to McDonald's, and in the play area a six-year-old kid said, "Get out of here, fat cow! You don't belong in here." The pediatrician suggested Health-Works!, which began by giving Clara a stress test to see if her heart and lungs could handle the workout program. After, the Lays met with a dietitian, psychologist, and nutritionist.

The Lays say they shop differently now, reading labels in the supermarket and veering toward the fruits and vegetable aisle first. They've changed the house, too, eliminating white sugar and the twelve-pack of soda the family used to imbibe regularly.

Alicia packs her daughter's lunch for school every day—also a new phenomenon. "Children live what they learn," she says with more than a tinge of regret. She actually blames herself for her daughter's weight problems. "The way I was feeding her was kind of neglectful. I had to realize that I'm Clara's mother and this home is what I'm supposed to be taking care of. It was like she was suffering for the consequences of the things *I* was choosing. So I had to rethink the things I was doing. I felt very guilty. It was like an epiphany that I was the one who was doing the grocery shopping and going through the drive-throughs. I don't think I did know better. I really wanted to reward them and so many times you choose food."

Clara no longer eats sugar, and gets a low-fat pudding in her lunch every other day, along with sugar-free Jell-O and fruit-flavored water. She plans her treats herself. "If she knows there's a wedding she will plan for it. 'Do I want the wedding cake or go to the ice cream store or what?' Now she looks ahead."

Clara has a trampoline, and she participates in gym, and she's on maintenance at the hospital, which means she and her family meet with a dietitian once a month. "One of my favorite things is getting to play games at the hospital," says Clara. "And the rewards to make me stay on the diet, like going to the movies, or bowling. It's fun."

Now Clara is harping on her mother's health. Alicia would like to lose weight herself. She's dropped about eight pounds now that she has incorporated Clara's meal plan into the family's, but she has another forty-two to go. It's hard; she drinks about two Cokes a day, although never in front of Clara.

"I want my mom to lose weight—a lot," Clara says. "And for her to stop smoking."

Alicia promised to stop on June 12. And she did—for a few weeks, until she started back up again.

» «

While hospital programs are better than fat camps—they involve the family, and at least they're run by medical professionals—they're not necessarily the answer, either. Once again, these programs illustrate the crucial point that losing weight requires enormous dedication, commitment, and motivation. While behavior modification might work for some people, it's certainly not for everyone. (It didn't work for me: The motivation to get thin never surpassed my immediate desire to eat—not for more than a few days, anyway.) It takes a lot of work to live and eat healthfully, and most importantly, it requires the desire. Without that, nothing works.

3

mothers against
fat kids

energetic, responsible parents who know they can't depend on the fat-camp solution, and don't feel like they need a hospital program to educate or structure them, have been known to take a revolutionary approach to their child's weight loss: They try to go it alone.

Like so many parents, Tammy Cohen and Deborah Frohlinger met through their kids. They had lots in common. They are both modern Orthodox Jews (which means that while they won't drive on the Sabbath and they're kosher, they will wear jeans and swear), they both have young kids, and, perhaps more important, they both have kids with weight problems. David, Tammy's ten-year-old son, is four foot ten and 120 pounds; Natalie, Deborah's eight-year-old, is in the 95th percentile in weight for her age group. The two women got to talking, and realized that with their combined expertise they could really do something. Deborah is an advertising VP who has worked on the Slim Fast account; Tammy has an MBA and is a total go-getter.

Right around the time they were hatching their idea, ABC's *The View* was holding auditions for "Meredith's Club," Meredith Vieira's earnest attempt to help overweight kids lose weight before a national TV audience. They would offer nutrition counseling, a shrink, and a fitness trainer for one year. It would be a win-win situation all around: The kids would lose weight, the ratings would shoot up (obesity, after all, is *hot*), and the shrink and nutritionist would get national publicity. Tammy's son David auditioned and was accepted. Tammy swooned.

Here's the thing about Tammy Cohen: She is the kind of person you want on your side. She probably had lots of friends at school. I imagine her as the ringleader, the one who came up with all the ideas for the rest of the gang to follow. She's smart as a whip, funny as hell, and good-looking, blonde and tall. Call her Erin Brockovichstein.

Tammy, who is diabetic, lives in a large apartment on the Upper East Side of Manhattan with her husband, Sydney, and three sons. Sydney is a big guy—maybe 240 pounds—but he's tall and wears his weight well. Their son David has always been a little chubby—not fat, just pudgy. If he grew a few feet—which he will—he'd be fine. The nutritionist at *The View* told him not to lose weight but not to gain. I keep wondering if this whole weight thing is going to make him nuts, if he will rebel later on in life and blow up. He shares a room with his younger brother, Aaron, who is eight and thin and adorable, and has won tons of chess trophies. I wonder if David is jealous of him.

Because Tammy is an innovator, and because she knows things don't happen unless someone instigates them, she and Deborah decided to start a program for kids and their parents who are grappling with weight issues. It would be called Kids in Control (KIC) and would offer six weeks of exercise for kids seven to twelve, twice a week. "These kids don't want to sit in a classroom—they want to run and play, move their bodies," she says in a thick Long Island accent.

As for mothers, they need a place where they can vent their feelings about being the parents of overweight kids, so while the kids worked out, the parents would learn nutrition and proper feeding techniques. "We're moms, we know our kids," says Tammy. "We're educated people. You don't necessarily need an expert telling you how to deal with your kids. Mothers can get together or a father who is concerned about his kids or an aunt and find a way to reach these kids. You don't need an expert to figure it out. You need to get together and work as a team. Look at Mothers Against Drunk Driving—there are so many mothers that said, 'I'm going to work on this and figure it out' and that's that we're trying to do."

To get KIC started, Tammy researched other programs to see what was out there. KIC is loosely modeled on two of the more popular programs: Kidshape, which was started in Los Angeles in 1987 by Dr. Naomi Neufeld, and ShapeDown, which was developed in 1979 by faculty members of the University of California, San Francisco, School of Medicine. Both are family-based weight management programs for children ages six to eighteen; registered dietitians teach the programs and behavior therapists work with participants on lifestyle changes in nutrition and physical activity. Meetings are held in churches, hospitals, and community centers, and costs run from $100 to $600 per session. Both programs are similar to La Rabida's Fit Matters—and most hospital programs, for that matter—in that family involvement is crucial.

Before you can even join ShapeDown, for example, you have to adhere to guidelines, which include, "Letting go of weightism and accepting your child's natural build; creating a light-but-not-depriving food environment at home; giving your child direct messages that you accept and value him or her; setting limits with your child and following through consistently; and being a good role model by improving your own weight, eating or inactivity problems." Parents are also required to attend all of the weekly two-and-a-half-hour sessions for ten weeks, and complete about an hour of reading a week and fifteen minutes of record keeping. And there is a caveat: If any family member doesn't bring his or her book and completed work to a session, no members of that family will be admitted.

Tammy has modified these programs, and she's trying to be realistic. "To us it's not a weight-loss or weight-management thing, it's a get-healthy thing for kids of all ages," she says. "You're going to learn what your body is about. It's going to help everybody down the road. We're giving them the opportunity to improve their whole body and their mind."

She also believes that the only people who can help are those who've been there, so she hopes to recruit mentors—older kids who've battled weight and succeeded—for the younger kids.

"It's like Scared Straight. They have these kids coming in and talking about their drug experiences. That's what we want to do."

Since signing up for *The View*, Tammy's son David has been trying to eat less and exercise more. He swims three times a week, and plays soccer on Sundays. And he's not shy about it. "My friends think it's cool that I'm on TV," he says. "I tell the other kids, 'When you eat, try to leave something over. Instead of candy, chew gum. Eat a lot of veggies so you stay healthy and confident.'" He wants to be twenty or thirty pounds less. He knows he's not obese, but he's pragmatic: "One hundred and twenty pounds at four foot ten isn't light for my age."

Tammy says she has seen changes in her son, even though she doesn't think *The View* is following through on its part. For one thing, the kids aren't accountable to anyone. The trainer is in Los Angeles, and the nutritionist only talks on the phone with her kid once a month. David never meets with her face-to-face. What good is that?

Still, David is learning. A few weeks ago, for example, his best friend, who is "handsome and thin," according to Tammy, stayed over. Tammy allotted three candies to both kids, and David went and picked out all sugar-free candy. "An hour later he wanted more—but that was my fault, because I shouldn't have left it sitting there," she says.

One afternoon in mid-October Tammy, Deborah, and I meet at the Prime Grill, a kosher restaurant in midtown Manhattan. The place is all atwitter. Madonna came in the night before with her kabbalah friends and everyone is still glowing from the sighting. The rumors fly: *She's practically Jewish—she's calling herself Esther! Soon she'll be one of us, for real!*

Tammy is talking animatedly about the weight thing; it's all she thinks about these days. A friend from Florida called her the other day to tell her that her son, Joshua, had lost fifteen pounds. "His mother said, 'He's tired of being teased. He's tired of having comments made to him. He came to me and said, 'Mom, what am I going to do? How do I go on a diet? What should I eat?'" Tammy recalls. "So she said, 'You know what Josh, there is no diet. Just eat half of what's on your plate. Eat whatever you want, just eat half of it and then between meals try not to eat anything. If you're really starving, have fruit in between.' That's how he lost fifteen pounds."

"Had he ever asked her before?" I ask.

"No."

Aha! I think. This is not a kid whose parents shamed him.

"Both of my kids have somewhat of a weight issue," says Deborah. She is nervous and frazzled, and slightly shrill. I imagine she's hard on her kids. Whereas Tammy is a force, Deborah seems easily stressed. "But I see a big difference between my boy and girl. My daughter has a relationship with food that is different from my son's. He's not going to cry or fight. If I say, 'No, you can't eat that,' she does. She has an emotional relationship with food."

Deborah and her husband have been harassing their daughter Natalie since she was three. When Natalie was in the first grade Deborah got a phone call from the school psychologist. "The first thing out of her mouth was, 'I'm concerned about her weight,'" Deborah recalls sadly.

So, they began working on it at home, serving healthy food and trying to exercise. But it was difficult. "All my husband and I were doing is running after her, 'No Natalie, no Natalie.' I put her on the scale every week. We've gone through terrible rebellion. She's told me she hates me and slams the door. It's horrible. I'm at the office sobbing. This poor child."

Well, duh, I want to say. *How do you think she's going to act?*

"You have to be creative and figure a way to do it so the kid feels like a partner in the process," says Tammy. "It's not about the parent telling the kid what to do and the kid doing it but it's about the parent and the kid having this relationship where they can work together. Like while you guys are watching TV get into a yoga position. How much fun would that be?"

"What about when he goes to school? You have no control over him there," I say. "He can eat whatever he wants."

David goes to a private Jewish day school, and Tammy is very upset about the lunch there. There's no one watching them, the kids can go up to the food line as many times as they want, and it's all junk—starches and carbs and fats. That's something she plans to address in the future.

And outside of school?

"It's everywhere," she acknowledges. "They have their own money. I say to them, 'I want you to be free and independent but you have to know the right choices to make. You have to know how to balance it.'"

"But what's the worst thing that could happen if your child is overweight if he's healthy and happy?" I ask. "What would be so bad? One woman I talked to said, 'I just see it as a failure. I see it as I have failed this child.' But if he's happy, you haven't failed. If he's healthy, you haven't failed. If he finds love, you haven't failed."

Tammy shakes her head adamantly. "If you went to the doctor and he said, 'Your blood test shows that you have very high cholesterol,' what are you going to do? You look good, you're thin, who cares if you have cholesterol and don't do anything about it? You're going to end up being sickly. It's the same thing with this. You're overweight, you don't eat properly, you shove the food in your mouth, you don't take a minute and you want to eat all the time. Let's work on this not because you're not a wonderful person and I don't love you madly but because as you get older you're going to go away to college and you're going to be with your friends. I'm not going to be there to tell you what to do!"

Tammy says she was a skinny kid, but as in many Jewish homes (and Italian and Greek and Russian and almost every other ethnic group), food played a huge role in hers. "My family only got along when we ate," she says with a laugh. "As a kid I ate whatever I wanted; when I got older I had no idea how to stop it. I wouldn't eat one yogurt, I'd eat five. One year I gained twenty-five pounds. My mother was like, 'What are you doing?' I remember thinking, 'I don't know how to control this.' When I was in high school I did the black beauties, the amphetamines, because everybody did that stuff, and then I couldn't maintain my weight-loss. It was very hard. I always felt like if I was twenty pounds thinner I'd be much happier."

Three months ago she had a revelation, and it came from a rather unlikely source: Suzanne Somers. Tammy swears by her program, Somersize. She maintains that it teaches people to be sensible with what they eat. It taught her. "I'm forty-one years old and now I'm finally getting control of my life," she says—a rather broad statement, considering she's only talking about food, but that's what food represents when you're not in control of it—your life.

Deborah never had a weight issue as a kid—she was a ballerina and danced three or four times a week. When she was sixteen her parents divorced and she gained weight. Her mother immediately put her on Weight Watchers; when Deborah had her kids at age twenty-eight, she weighed 118 pounds. Today, she's about thirty pounds overweight, which annoys her.

Both women agree that the real issue is that there's nowhere for the parents of overweight kids to go, and no place for fat kids to be around other fat kids, besides fat camp. There are no support groups, no online chat rooms.

Tammy feels the problem extends to the so-called experts, too. "None of them was willing to help me with my child's issue," she says. "They don't know how."

"Less than a third of all U.S. medical schools have a required nutrition course," says Dr. Steven Zeisel, chair of the Department of Nutrition at the University of North Carolina, Chapel Hill. While many schools do try to incorporate nutrition as part of other course material, few instructors actually review practical techniques.

An August 2003 report from the American Academy of Pediatrics, an organization of 60,000 pediatricians, recommended members make obesity screening and counseling part of children's regular checkups. The academy also offered eight suggestions for how doctors can intervene with patients before weight problems begin—including paying attention to individual risk factors for obesity and monitoring kids at high risk (that is, babies with high birth weights and formula-fed babies, as well as children living in single-parent homes; children who spend too much time in front of the TV; and those with parents who are somewhat obsessed with their children's diets). It also suggests tracking body mass indexes. Parents are advised to be more aware of eating arrangements and patterns, keeping children busy and alert, and minimizing their exposure to TV and video games.

The report is important but insufficient, says Dr. William Dietz, director of the division of nutrition and physical activity at the Centers for Disease Control and Prevention (CDC) National Center for Chronic Disease Prevention and Health Promotions. "It tells pediatricians a lot about what they should be assessing and what they should focus on in terms of preventative or therapeutic efforts. The missing piece is, 'How do you actually do it?' And that's the key question. How do you engage families? It takes a different type of training to change behavior than pediatricians are receiving in medical school."

It's a good question, and an important one. How *do* you engage families in a positive, constructive way? That's something Deborah and Tammy are actively trying to figure out.

"I don't want to put her in therapy, but maybe I should," Deborah says of her daughter. "As a mother, I don't know what to do. My husband would starve my children if he could. He's even stricter than I am about this."

"Yeah, and that's what's hard," says Tammy. "The parents have to be unified. That's the way you have a family commitment."

"But you have to start this from day one," I point out. "You can't suddenly change the rules when they're twelve years old. They're not going to listen to you."

"Do you think part of it is that parents have become more permissive in general?" Tammy asks. "With parenting, I think the issue is limits. We have to give limits with food. Kids need structure. I see two-year-old kids negotiating with their parents. What are you negotiating? Pick them up and put them in the carriage!"

"I have all my kids' friends at my house and I tell them, 'If you want to eat you have to eat at the table,'" says Deborah. "There are limits in life. Kids think things are negotiable and they're not."

"What happens if they don't lose weight? Can you accept your child overweight?" I ask.

"Of course I will accept it, but I expect her to take control of the situation," Deborah says. "My disappointment would be in the fact she is not taking control."

"Would you be disappointed in her or in you?"

"I think at that age more her. She can take control of things in her life. But I say to myself, 'How can I expect her to lose weight when I get on the scale and I haven't lost weight?'"

"I could totally accept David if he were fifteen, twenty pounds overweight because I've been battling that my whole life," says Tammy. "I can't accept him if he's fifty pounds overweight. I would have a really hard time with him if he were obese. I'm not going to lie about it. Because of the health issues, because of everything. There is no reason to be like that. I don't care how happy you are; it's not okay."

Besides, she adds, he should be grateful. "He's got supportive parents and resources at his fingertips. I would be pissed off that he can't even seem to appreciate that. I know it sounds harsh, but I'm trying to give him the advantage of doing something and gaining control over his life so this doesn't become a 250-pound problem."

The good news is that by osmosis her other kids are picking up the good habits, she says (or, I might say but don't, they may have picked up different genetics at birth). "My middle son, Aaron, has a totally different mindset. He's athletic. He's a shy kid but friends with the world. He heard me talking about this thing and he started listening and he was like, 'I want to do that.' He'll give up the candy if he thinks it's going to put him in the next pound level. He's like that.

"With my oldest son everything came easy, like being smart in school, but Aaron had to work for it. Thank God he had motivation. David doesn't have motivation. David has motivation to buy the latest gadget, but he doesn't have the motivation to not eat that candy."

"That comes from within," I say. "You can't instill that in some-body, can you?"

"My youngest son is going to eat healthy because he doesn't have a choice. He's not going to know any other way," she says. "Now he's eating broccoli and things I wasn't feeding the kids before. He's got a sweet tooth but he's three and he's not going to love me less be-cause I'm not giving him candy. With David I've been a really per-missive mom, giving him whatever he wants. He was my firstborn and if he wanted candy I gave him candy. If he wanted to go back to the dinner table he went back to the dinner table. It made it easier getting him out of the house and easier getting him to school be-cause he was always defiant and gave me a hard time. So I gave in and I gave him lots of bad things and food was always a reward, as it was for me as a child. If I got hurt my mother would always give me something to eat. I did the same thing with him."

» «

Part of KIC's beauty is that it offers a monthly forum for women to voice their frustrations and ask questions and get insight from other women who are raising overweight—or perceived as over-weight—kids. Call it Mothers Against Fat Kids.

The first meeting is on a frosty October night. Eight women show up, plus Tammy and Deborah, and gather in a vacant room at the LA Sports Club, a swanky gym on the Upper East Side. Some are a little heavy, but they're certainly not fat—though they all seem to have food issues. They are all white, mostly Jewish, and there are no men present.

I have invited a seventeen-year-old boy named Lawrence Capici, who has weighed as much as 322 pounds, to sit in. Lawrence and his mother, Rhonda, have searched high and low for support groups for obese kids and their parents. I thought this might fit some kind of bill, though as time goes on it's clear it doesn't. Lawrence was seri-ously obese, while these mothers have kids who are thirty pounds overweight, tops. Lawrence is their worst nightmare.

Tammy opens the discussion, introducing herself and explaining the situation with her son. "There's nowhere to go to vent," she says. "You don't need to be judged as a parent by anyone."

Deborah cries about Natalie, especially when she retells a story. "Before she went to the beach one day over the summer, I screamed at her, 'Look at yourself in that bathing suit!' Yet, I do not control myself."

Lawrence is shy and quiet. He doesn't smile at all. Instead, his mother speaks. "There's nothing in Manhattan for overweight kids—only anorexic girls and boys." As the mother of a truly obese child, she was clearly out of sorts.

Finally Lawrence speaks up, so softly that the women sit forward in their seats to hear better. "My parents were trying to help me my entire life—it seemed like they were always trying something new for me," he says. "Sometimes I wanted to do it and sometimes I wasn't into it. But you don't need to keep telling the kids that they're fat. They know it already."

I look around the room. The mothers nod wordlessly. Apparently this has never occurred to them before.

Lisa has three boys. One is slightly overweight: five feet tall and 110 pounds. Michelle has four kids; two are skinny, two are heavy. Her four-year-old weighs the same as the six-and-a-half–year-old. He wears a size 7. Miriam's daughter is in the second grade. She's heavy and "doesn't make the right choices. How do I get her to make the right choices?"

Andrea, who is big herself, has four kids. Her son, Michael, is nine, and 140 pounds. He is very developmentally advanced for his age. The other day she started crying because she found pubic hair on him. They are going to an endocrinologist to see why he is developing so early.

A woman named Danalee Wechsler pipes up. Danalee is thirty-seven and a pediatric occupational therapist who lives on the Upper East Side. She is the daughter of Holocaust survivors; both of her parents were in Auschwitz, and her whole family is heavy. "My sister is over 200 pounds, and I fluctuate fifty pounds up, sixty pounds down, like an accordion," she says. She is not a parent, but she says she's interested in not screwing up the kids she may one day have. As someone who has lost and gained hundreds of pounds, she knows what it's like to be obsessed.

"We mess up our children with so many different things, this is just one less thing I wanna screw them up with," she says. "I'm still not married; I have so much time to work on myself cognitively, emotionally, I would just like to make my kids as healthy as I can. Weight is something I've struggled with. If they're going to be over-weight it's in the gene pool. I just don't have to have them obsess over it; I'd like to make them as healthy as possible emotionally and mentally. If I give them fat thighs, hopefully I'll have money to give them liposuction."

The most upsetting person in the room to me is Lorraine Evans, a southern flower with two kids and a chef for a husband. Their four-year-old son is not overweight, but the five-year-old, Livia, is three feet nine inches and fifty-one pounds. Lorraine hides snacks—often Fritos—for her son; everything in her daughter's lunch box is monitored. "Then I eat them and hope I don't have Frito breath," she admits, noting that she always had weight prob-lems. "On my thirteenth birthday my mother bought me a scale. But I look back and I was not that heavy.

"My daughter will say, 'Do I look thin?' I'll say, 'It's not a fat or thin issue. It's looking in the mirror and knowing you're beautiful inside and out.' But then she hears me going, 'Mommy's as fat as a house.'" She wonders aloud why her daughter cannot control her appetite.

I have been digging my nails into my palms so as not to open my big mouth, but finally I can't help myself. "What makes *you* not able to control *your* appetite?" I ask.

"I'm a stress eater; my daughter's not," she says. "She has no stress. She's five!"

"Maybe she does and you just don't know it," I respond. "Maybe she picks up on everything in your world." Lorraine looks utterly bewildered.

Clearly, these mothers aren't addressing the emotional component to their child's weight problems. Parents often have no idea what's in their kids' minds. They forget what it was like to be young, with problems and yes, even stresses, of their own. These stresses only grow bigger as they get older.

Ellyn Satter, a Madison, Wisconsin-based dietitian and the author of three books on feeding children, including *How to Get Your Kid to Eat—But Not Too Much* (Bell Publishing, 1987), notes that "Children can overeat—or underexercise—because they're stressed. Children are stressed when parents are too busy and don't take much interest in them; children are stressed when parents are so overburdened by life circumstances that they can't keep them safe. . . . Finally, children often overeat because they are afraid they aren't going to get enough to eat. Children who live day after day with food insecurity eat as much as they can get, when they can get it. Children whose parents limit their food intake for fear they will get fat do the same. Children whose food intake is restricted tend to get fatter, not thinner, as they get older." The ultimate paradox! You're damned no matter what you do!

Helen has five kids of varying shapes and sizes. One of her kids went to Camp Shane three times. He lost twenty-seven pounds the first year, which he promptly gained back when he came home. The second year he returned to camp and embraced his inner entrepreneur: "He sold shirts to counselors and kids, or traded them for food," she says. "The counselors thought it was funny." He lost twenty-one pounds the second year, which he also gained back. The third year, his bar mitzvah year, he lost forty pounds, which he's kept off so far.

Helen took him to a nutritionist, who handed him plastic food and asked him to show her what he ate. "The kid makes a beautiful picture of fruits and vegetables and meat and eggs, but that's not what he eats!" she says with a laugh. "But he knows what she wants to hear."

The mothers make me so angry. I feel like I have regressed to adolescence. They obviously love their kids and worry about them, but they have their own stuff to deal with. It's not so much their lack of self-control I find so irksome, but their lack of self-knowledge, that they're not looking at their own roles in creating the problem (with the exception of Tammy). Parents have to lead by example, from day one. If they can't curb their own desires then how can they expect their kids to? And I can't help but wonder how big these kids really are. I look over at Lawrence Capici's mother, who had a 322-pound kid to deal with. How must she be feeling right now?

Instead of sympathizing with them—I'm probably close to their age—I feel like an obstinate kid: Hey, no one told you to reproduce. No one said it would be easy. Have you forgotten what it's like to be a kid?

These women are overlooking the emotional, physical, and medical reasons kids overeat. Plus, their kids don't seem to be obese—chubby, perhaps, but hardly fat.

When it's my turn to share, I say, "I'm Abby, and I'm writing a book on childhood obesity, and when I was twelve and gained twenty pounds my grandmother wouldn't let me visit her in Florida. I hear you guys talking and I just want to say, 'Shut up!' You're ruining your kids! You're gonna drive them bananas."

All eyes turn my way. They are not pleased. "You're not a parent," one says pointedly.

"No, I'm not. But I was a kid, and I'm still someone's kid. And when one of you says that you're sneaking Fritos and hoping that your daughter won't notice your Frito breath, well, what kind of message are you sending your kid? Kids are not stupid. It doesn't matter so much what you say—what you *think* sends the message all by itself. And kids know exactly what you're thinking." I still know, for example, when my mother disapproves of my appearance; I can tell the minute she walks into my house. She doesn't have to utter a word. I can see the way her eye imperceptibly traces my appearance. If she's pleased, she'll tell me I'm beautiful and that my figure is great. If not, she'll say nothing, but her internal sigh comes through loud and clear.

And then I think, okay, parenting is the hardest job in the world. These women are doing their best. They're trying to prevent their kids from becoming obese, they're trying to nip the problem in the bud before it becomes a bigger problem. What should they do— step in, or let the kid become 200 pounds and wait for the child to come to them for help? And how do you not drive your kid to the opposite end of the spectrum and create some kind of eating disorder?

In her book *Rescuing the Emotional Lives of Our Overweight Children* (Rodale, 2004), Sylvia Rimm acknowledges that parents who were overweight kids and are now in control of their weight tend to be very judgmental of their children. Consequently, they often end up micromanaging. "Parents need to be coaches instead of judges," she adds. "Good coaches are enthusiastic, positive and concerned. They convey a sense that they believe in the kids they coach. When you're a coach, you believe your children will do their best and they know it."

She's right. But that's a lot easier to say than do. Even experts can be baffled when it comes to their own families. Anne Fletcher, the dietitian and author of *Thin for Life,* spent a long time beating herself up for the weight her son Wes held onto for many years. Wes weighed 270 in eleventh grade, but finally lost weight on his own, without any prodding from her.

"You can't have me as a mother and not have food be an issue," she says. "I think I made it more of an issue than I wanted to, not with what I said but how I said it. Wes is also a child who has authority issues, not just with food but at school. What better way to get back at your parents?"

Fletcher's middle child, Tyler, is seventeen, naturally lean, and not interested in junk food. But her ten-year-old daughter is just starting to gain weight, and despite all Fletcher's expertise and all her experience with her son, she still doesn't know what to do.

» «

Meeting two: Wednesday, December 7, 2003.

It's a cold night, rainy and snowy. I have arranged for Rebecca Ross and Bryan Morris to come in. Rebecca and Bryan are both sixteen years old and very articulate ex-Camp Shaners. I thought it would be interesting for the mothers to hear their opinions. The kids are excited; they can't wait to tell parents what they really think the problem is: them! And they hope to help the parents answer the all-encompassing question, What do we do?

Bryan is adorable: black hair, blue eyes, and only slightly pudgy. He wears sneakers, a sweat jacket, gray shirt, and jeans, the high school–student uniform du jour. Rebecca has a round face and is big, but not huge. She is very pretty, with big eyes and clear skin. She wears clogs, jeans, white shirt; her straight hair is parted down the middle of her forehead. She is very theatrical. "I'm an actress," she says with a dramatic flourish. The gym's dietitian, Sydney Foster, is also here; KIC is one of her pet projects. She's not a therapist, though, which means she's not especially qualified to deal with all of the emotional, psychological, medical, and addictive components unique to obesity. But then, these mothers aren't really interested in all of that. They're looking for practical, quick solutions.

Deborah introduces herself first and talks about her kids. She says that after hearing Lawrence Capici at the last meeting, she changed her approach to her daughter. Now, she says, she tries to help keep herself in check and not focus so much on her kid.

Rebecca sees this as her chance to break in. She thinks the mothers are obsessing about nothing. "Your kids are so young, and none seem to be especially fat," she says.

"Even though the kids are under ten, there's only a limited time you have to start learning," the dietitian explains.

"I struggled all my life," says Lorraine, the Frito-sneaking mother. "It's a lot more emotional and painful at eleven and twelve than at five or six. My daughter just said that one of the kids told her she was the fattest kid in the class. I asked how it made her feel and she said, 'Oh, okay.' I want to help her with this so it doesn't get more painful."

Tammy pipes up. "My son says, 'I can't control myself. I want to eat all the time.' I said, 'What's going to happen if you don't eat?

You think you're going to pass out?' He got it. He just likes the idea of eating all the time."

Rebecca breaks in. "If the act of eating helps him, just give him less. Take less of the orange. Or a little clementine. I just found out fifty-one Goldfish is one serving." She looks very pleased with herself for this, and the mothers laugh.

"My biggest challenge is quantity and portion control," says Lorraine. "Right now we're trying to see about tennis for my daughter. It's about $500 and my husband is complaining. Meanwhile, I always say the wrong thing to my kids. I've said to my daughter, 'Do you want your clothes to fit?' I find myself screaming at 8 P.M., 'Eating is over, the kitchen is closed!' A nutritionist told me that my daughter is eating adult-sized portions."

"I control the portions at home but not when she goes to a friend's house," Lorraine continues. "My husband phones ahead and tells the person to please watch what she eats. It's horrible, but what else can we do? I call up the moms and say, 'Can you feed her healthy food?'"

"I don't think that's so wrong," says Deborah.

Helen does. "I had one mother say to me, 'I watched what he ate,'" she says. She is very matter-of-fact, like Tammy, and she pulls no punches. "I didn't ask anyone to watch him or see if he can have an extra piece of cake. It was an extra zinger."

Tammy nods vigorously. "I let my son stay at my friend's house," she says. "She knows what he's doing and she gave him three Krispy Kremes for breakfast. He came home and told me, and I saw that as a victory, even though he ate it."

"In a perfect world he wouldn't eat it at all," Rebecca points out. She's right, but how realistic is it to expect children to decline some of the most delectable confections ever put on this earth?

Harriet wears tight jeans, chic black patent-leather boots, a black shirt, and woolen beret. She is, by far, the hippest one in the room, and the thinnest. But she is also whacked about food. "I was on a diet at twelve. I'm forty-six, and I still have issues with food. My mother would call other mothers and say, 'My daughter is fat.' I'm a product of that neurosis. I never wanted to make food an issue for my daughter. She's ten and a little chubby. I don't want this to affect her for the rest of her life. It can make you insane."

"Do you pick your battles?" asks Lila. "Do I say, yeah, you can have popcorn but with no butter? Do I let her have a Mountain Dew or Diet Coke and fry her brain on chemicals?"

Rebecca has been holding up her hand the whole time. She looks pained, as if not speaking up is killing her.

"I think 'No' is the worst word. If you say no it's going to make the child want to eat. If you show her a healthy eating style eventually she'll adopt it as her own."

"Good point," says Sydney.

She hands out papers and the group reads them aloud like fragments of the Bible:

Put your fork down between bites.

Take a sip of water after each bite.

Start dinner with a salad and include veggies in the main course.

Do not snack or eat in front of the TV.

When you have a snack or meal, take out your portion before eating it (for example, put your pretzels in a bowl rather than eat out of the bag).

Always ask yourself: "Am I eating because I'm hungry or because I'm bored?"

Eat slowly.

When you want to snack, go for low-calorie, high-nutrient food choices like fruit or cut veggies or skim dairy.

Drink plenty of water throughout the day, especially at meal times.

Discourage weight-loss shortcuts like fasting, fad diets (including low-carb diets), crash dieting, diet pills.

Reward hard work with new music or a new book rather than with food.

Fill afterschool time with physical activities: music, drama, sports, or visiting friends rather than snacking or playing video games or watching TV.

Then she hands out a worksheet, a "Behavior change commitment" form that each kid is supposed to fill out, along with his concerns (for example, that he might eat too many sweets after dinner when he's not hungry) and goals (for example, consuming enough food during the day so he doesn't overdo it at night).

The next section has an area for kids to write down the steps they can take to help them achieve their goal.

The child is supposed to check how many of these goals he has accomplished, and how often. All in all, not so dissimilar from the folks at La Rabida—and just as difficult to achieve. It's all good advice, but I can't help wondering—and I know Bryan and Rebecca are thinking the same thing—*What will happen to these kids once they're out of their parents' jurisdiction?* It's easier to tell smaller kids what to do; it's a different story with a grumpy adolescent.

Bryan is not impressed, and why should he be? He's a teenager. It's his job to go against his parents. This kind of thing only irritates him, provoking an emotional response about rebellion, condescension, and patronization. He glances down at the piece of paper and makes a face. "I would never sign anything like this," he says. "I hate commitment."

"I'm not saying you're committing to losing five pounds, just to changing something," says Sydney, who's visibly annoyed with the kids' interruptions. "For whatever reason, when people have to sign something it makes it more real."

"I'd feel horrible if I didn't do it. Then I might as well have two Smart Ones," says Rebecca, referring to the highly addictive Weight Watchers frozen treats.

Lorraine agrees with Rebecca. "I would never put this paper in front of my five-year-old. This is all for me, so I can have the intelligence. The last thing I want her to think is that there's something wrong with her."

"I went through the diet plan with my kid and put it on the fridge," says Deborah. "It put her more in control."

"What are the triggers that cause your kids to be out of control?" asks Sydney.

"My daughter asks, 'When will I lose weight?' Then she eats and eats," says Lorraine. "What's the issue when a child is full and they look at a cabinet for the ginger snaps or whatever? What do you do about that?"

"Chew ten times. Sip water," says Rebecca. "Do any of you make your kids finish everything on their plates?"

Maternal chorus: NO!

"Just checking." The mothers laugh.

"Kids mirror us," Lila says. "We have to change the way we are. It's a twofold process." *At last! Progress!*

Sydney the dietitian offers another homework assignment. She wants their kids to write down three questions they have about food, nutrition, weight loss, hunger, calories, exercise, and dieting. "And if you think doing the behavioral change will be detrimental, don't do it."

» «

Bryan and Rebecca are less than thrilled with the meeting. The mothers seemed horribly unaware of the difference between constructive and nonconstructive assistance, and more likely to create more problems than to help their kids. I identify with Bryan and Rebecca; they make some valid points. What struck me most, though, is how much they wanted to be heard.

Bryan is fuming. "God help those poor children!"

"I was ready to scream at them!" says Rebecca.

"At this rate," says Bryan, "they have not touched the problem."

"Okay," I say to Bryan and Rebecca. "But don't you give them credit for at least trying to fix the problem now?"

"My mom created my self-esteem issue," says Rebecca. "I wasn't fat until my mom told me I was. My parents started bugging me about my weight before my bat mitzvah. I remember wearing my dress and they said, 'Oh, you need to lose weight.' The way they went about it was, 'You look horrible.' My dad would joke about it—when we were kids my dad would call my brother 'Half Pint' and me 'Full Pint.'"

Bryan picks up the commitment form and waves it. "I wanted to say, 'Please burn this.' If these parents were blind, there wouldn't be any problems."

"If you overeat for subconscious reasons, why shouldn't your slowing down of eating be subconscious?" he continues. "The more freedom you trust your children with, the better they're going to be able to handle it. The first place a kid should have freedom is in the house."

Yes, I think. And no. It's like the question many of my friends have about smoking pot: Is it better for a parent to let the kid get stoned in front of them, or should they do it behind their backs? My mother once asked me not to eat a piece of pie in front of her. She didn't want to witness my destruction. This, of course, propelled me to hide food, which wasn't any better.

"When we were at my house my mom was eating the Halloween candy under a blanket. I heard it," says Bryan. "My mother would order pizzas for my thin brother and not for me."

"With these kids, say, 'We'll be there for you. We won't push you. When you're ready, come to us,'" says Rebecca.

Their ideas are rushing out in a torrent and they're not answering my main question. So I ask again. "What's the best way to stop a chubby child from becoming an obese one, without driving him mad? What should a parent do after he or she has screwed up?"

Bryan looks me straight in the eye. "Nothing," he says. "You're doomed."

» «

He's right, in a way. After a certain age, when kids have minds of their own and the ability to buy food where they want, there's not much the parent can do until the kid is ready himself. Conversely, without early intervention, fat children are very likely to grow into fat adults—which is precisely Tammy's point.

Ellyn Satter has spent years thinking about this very issue. Satter's mission is to develop what she calls "eating competency" in children, which involves teaching kids to love food and teaching parents to encourage their children's self-sufficiency. Parents decide "what, when and where" their children eat; their children decide "how much and whether" they will eat. Snacks and junk food aren't withheld—they're just not around, period. Theoretically, over time children will learn how to moderate their own food consumption.

Her approach makes sense, but of course it's most effective if you follow her guidelines from day one (she works with kids from two months through adulthood.) For a parent who didn't know about Satter and now has a severely overweight twelve-year-old, she suggests a secondary intervention, which includes a reexamination of the child's medical history since birth, a nutritional breakdown of her eating patterns over a week, office consultations, and a videotaped analysis of a series of family meals. Satter explores whether the weight gain is a passing phase, and asks questions like, "Is the family following her suggestion about the division of responsibility? Are they withholding food from the child? Are family problems leading the child to seek edible solace?"

Satter has seen success using this approach with older kids, though she admits it's difficult trying to get an already angry teenager to collaborate. But it's not impossible.

"I worked with a twelve-year-old who was upset about his weight," Satter told me. "He wanted to go out for football and couldn't run as fast as the other kids. There was room for improvement. We worked on it together. With older children it *has* to be their idea and they have to ask for their parents' help."

And what about kids who ask for help one day and then resent it the next? (I often did this. When I was thirteen I spent a weekend at a friend's house and made sure her mother knew, in advance, that I was on a diet. Her mom prepared special meals for me, which I happily ate—in addition to the same regular food as my friend who wasn't on the diet. She later informed her mother of this, who, in turn, was visibly annoyed that she'd wasted all that time cooking for me when I wasn't serious about dieting.)

The first thing the parents have to do is look at themselves, Satter says. Why is the child so vulnerable to the food? "A lot of things can happen that can make kids too fat—being too controlling is one of them," she says. "Restricting food intake whereupon they become obsessed with food. Being inconsistent about feeding them is another. Children really do need their parents to attend to feeding them, to pay attention to meal time and getting the family together and being present with the child at meal time."

This reminds me of Lisa Williams, whose nine-year-old daughter, Kate, is slowly developing a weight problem. One night Kate broke down because she was so unhappy about what she weighed and worried she would become as big as her sister, Emily, who weighs 250. She begged her mother to help. "Okay," Lisa said.

"You always say that but then you never do," Kate said, through tears.

Together, they went to the fridge and ceremoniously tossed out a carton of Healthy Choice low-fat ice cream. "Yes, it was Healthy Choice and only a quarter of the calories of Häagen-Dazs," Williams explained. "But in my house, none of us is really good about portion control, or the 'occasional treat' idea. First, whoever eats half a cup of ice cream? And second, if it's in the house at all, we'll eat it every night until it's gone, and then I'll buy another.

"Because my own parents were so controlling—my dad was obese as a kid and obsessed that his kids would be, too—I went the opposite way with my kids and didn't regulate them at all," Lisa confesses. "I worried about making them feel deprived. But I guess I went too far. Really, *I'm* the one who still feels deprived about ice cream. Kate feels deprived of more guidance." In the ensuing weeks, Kate lost two pounds and has maintained her interest in healthier eating.

Kids need—nay, crave—structure. They want to be told what to do, at least when they're young. They want their parents to be, well, parents—not to shame them, not to judge them, not to condemn them because of their weight, but to love them, flaws and all. "Parents have to do their jobs; it's not wise to just leave the child to their

own devices with eating," says Satter. "Maintain a division of responsibility in feeding. Maintain the structure of meals and snacks
and at mealtime offer a variety of food: a main dish, a couple of
carbs like bread and potatoes or rice, fruit and vegetables, milk is
important—and dessert.

"If a child is insulin resistant or has high cholesterol, in ninety-
nine out of a hundred cases there's room for improvement with respect to the way feeding is conducted and one can optimize
feeding—snacks, not letting kids graze—by turning off the TV set
and letting kids get bored enough so they find something else to do.
For most kids that represents an enormous improvement in their
eating activity and physical health. So there's a great deal that can
be done before you go anywhere close to a weight-reduction diet."

» «

Meeting 3: January 2004.

Manhattan is in the midst of a hellacious winter: freezing ice,
sleet, and snow, on a daily basis. Tonight only four women show up
to the meeting, along with Sydney the dietitian and Dr. Palmo
Pasquariello, Tammy's pediatrician. Tonight's agenda: new diet
strategies.

Sydney asks about the commitments from last time. How did
they go? Have they been at all successful? Were the kids able to
stick to them? Were *they?*

Not really. Tammy has just returned from a vacation in Aruba.
"We ate like pigs," she says with a laugh. "We went insane, like we'd
been let out of a cage. David ate ice cream, he drank Coke, not Diet
Coke. I was eating French fries and my kids were like, 'You're not
supposed to be eating that.' I was like, 'Shut up.' But now I know
what it's like to be nagged."

Still, there was some success. "David's commitment was, 'I do
not want to eat snacks when I'm bored,'" says Tammy. "He said,
'Let's think about what I can eat for dinner.' We wrote down a meal
plan. He likes knowing what to expect and *he* came up with what to

do. I hung it up in the kitchen." David, clearly, is involved. He has grown and is still the same size he was a year ago. Victory!

"My son has his hands in the cereal box—I smacked his hands and put them in the sink and gave him two fruits," says Lila.

The women then debate what kind of cereal is okay: Multigrain? Cheerios? Special K?

Special K with Splenda, Sydney says.

"But what about chemicals? Is Splenda really good for you?" I ask.

One woman, who has obviously been watching way too much television, dramatically intejects: "But obesity kills."

What about kids who don't want to eat in the morning?

"If they're not hungry in the morning then they're eating too much the night before," says Sydney. She gets into some semantics. Breakfast is break the fast. Get it?

The women are over the moon with that one. Wowee! Who knew?

She offers vacation tips: Don't go to a hotel or on a cruise that has three meals a day included in the price—common sense, if you ask me. How could it not be? Don't take your kids to a buffet if they have a food problem!

This all seems like big news to the moms. I'm just constantly amazed at how unaware they are.

No one knows unaware parents better than Christina Houghton. Now fifty-three and an office manager at a law firm in Manhattan, Houghton has been obese her whole life. She is still obese—300 pounds now—although she's recently down from 400, which she sees as a huge victory (and it is). She and her husband, David, who has adult-onset diabetes and is about fifty pounds overweight, have one son, Mitchell, who is fourteen and on his way to obesity. He has gone to Camp Kingsmont for two years, but it hasn't worked.

Since Houghton was terrorized by her parents about her weight, she refuses to do that to Mitch. So what is she left with? A fourteen-year-old kid who is on his way to becoming obese—but one who knows his parents love, and more importantly, *get* him.

"It has been nothing but a struggle to help him develop healthy eating habits," she says. "I've always found myself being extra careful about not making him feel bad about himself for his tendency to overeat and his inability to make healthy food choices. We have joked for years that he is a 'dairytarian' and a 'carboholic.' For a long time I fought with him over his food choices. It got to the point where every meal was a battle. It was dreadful to deal with the constant arguing and I eventually gave up the fight.

"In my efforts to help Mitch change his diet I routinely have fresh fruits and vegetables in the house. He will not consider even touching vegetables and he is quite fussy about what fruit he will eat. Mitchell is well informed about diet and nutrition and he knows what he needs to eat for a healthier lifestyle. We all do our own swallowing and I need to believe that he will find a way to take better care of himself. At this point, all I can do is set a good example for him and I am committed to doing that. I have been working for years to undo the damage that was done to me—by my parents, my classmates, society, and myself. I constantly struggle with accepting myself for who I am rather than who I think I should be—or what society dictates is 'acceptable.' My biggest challenge as an obese woman has been to find a way to exercise and take better care of myself. Using the locker room at the YMCA has been the most significant accomplishment of my life thus far. After all these years, I am learning to appreciate my body and I am no longer ashamed of it."

Tammy and the rest of the moms might think she is being irresponsible, letting Mitch figure out the food thing on his own, but her point, to me, is clear: Why harangue her son when the rest of the world will happily do it for her? Why make him feel awful when he's assaulted with that on a daily basis? If anyone knows about the lasting damage peers, classmates, and society—but especially parents—do to overweight kids, it's she. And in her quest to reparent herself, she has discovered how to be a better parent to Mitch.

Her own past is telling: "At sixteen, when I got my driver's license, I was liberated and able to go anywhere I wanted," Houghton says. "The drive-through phenomenon was just beginning and

Dixie Cream Doughnuts was on the forefront of the new craze. I thought that the drive-through at the doughnut shop was a gift from God. I loved it. On countless occasions I would drive up and get exactly the kind of doughnuts I wanted.

"The drive-through didn't have a display case, so a person had to be an experienced buyer in order to purchase doughnuts at the window. I guess you'd be okay if you wanted a standard doughnut, like glazed or frosted or perhaps éclairs, but if you wanted something a little fancier, you needed to know the exact name of the product.

"My favorite doughnuts were long johns. Long johns were long rectangular custard-filled confections drenched in powdered sugar. They were messy as hell to eat, but they were really tasty. My second favorite were boston cream doughnuts. Cream-filled delights (not to be confused with custard) that were dunked in rich chocolate frosting. An exquisite treat. Rounding out my top three favorites were cinnamon buns. Cinnamon buns were fun to eat because you could unwind them as you ate them. They were also a great value because even though they were the same price as the other doughnuts, they were substantially larger. Generally, I could buy half a dozen doughnuts for only seventy-five cents and that was a good deal for high-quality doughnuts.

"Several times a week, whenever I had the car and a flimsy excuse to leave the house, I would cruise up to the Dixie Cream Doughnut window and get streamlined service. After I made my purchase, I would drive two blocks to the parking lot of the Presbyterian Church, let the engine idle and dive into the bag of delights. I remember frantically brushing every trace of powdered sugar off of my clothing when I finished my treats.

"Whenever I returned home from an excursion, my mother would interrogate me. She never asked me where I went, whom I saw, or what I did. She always wanted to know what I had eaten. Of course, I lied. It didn't make any difference what I had eaten, I denied everything. I don't know why she thought for a moment that I would admit to doing exactly what she didn't want me to do. I never talked to my parents about anything. I'm sure that this drove them crazy. I was a teenager. It was my responsibility to give them as hard a time as they were giving me. As far as I was concerned, what I ate was none of their business. It was my secret and I intended to keep it no matter what.

"One day, after a sumptuous, secretive time at Dixie Cream Doughnuts, I came home to a particularly intense interrogation. If my mother asked me once if I had eaten anything since lunchtime, she asked me at least five times. "Are you sure you haven't had anything to eat this afternoon? Nothing at all?" I denied having eaten anything. It was dinnertime and my mother wanted to know if I was hungry. Of course, I said. I always wanted to eat, regardless of whether I was hungry or not.

"My younger sister and older brother were both at home, and I set the table for dinner. My mother had a great recipe for Swiss Steak with tomatoes and onions. Served over mashed potatoes with green beans, it was one of my favorite meals. As she stood by the stove and dished up the plates, she directed me to put them on the table: "This is for Dad. Here's your brother's plate. This one is for your sister, and I'll take this one." Bewildered, I looked at my mother and pointed out that she had failed to dish up a plate for me. As I sat down at the table with my brother and sister, my mother glared at me and told me that my father had dished up my plate already. In a terse tone, she called my dad and told him to come to the table.

"My father rounded the corner from the family room carrying a large platter. A towering pyramid of at least two dozen doughnuts were stacked neatly on the dish. High atop the pyramid was a small carefully lettered pennant that read: Dixie Cream Doughnuts. I stared at the platter in disbelief and my parents stared at me. My brother seemed to be getting an immense amount of pleasure out of watching the entire scene unfold. I don't remember speaking. I only remember the tears as they welled in my eyes and streamed down my cheeks. I wanted to flee from the table but I was restrained by my mother's words: 'Since you enjoy eating doughnuts so much, you can have doughnuts for dinner.'

"I remained mute, too humbled to speak. I silently listened as my mother told me how she found out about my afternoon trip to the Dixie Cream Doughnut shop. My brother had told her that he had seen me there on his way home from school. To make it look like he wasn't ratting me out, he asked my mother if we were having doughnuts for dessert. He knew that we weren't and he also knew that he had caught me red-handed. I believe that sacrificing me to my parents was an indulgence too good for him to resist. By this time in his life, he had witnessed several years of my parents' determination to have an impact on my eating habits. Their annoyance and frustration with me had a significant impact on the entire family.

"I maintained my silence when my mother asked me why I wasn't eating my dinner. 'I thought you liked doughnuts, go ahead and eat them.' I couldn't stop crying. I wished that my tears would dissolve my body. I wanted to ask them how they could treat me this way, but I couldn't find the words. As they triumphantly started to eat their Swiss Steak and potatoes, I bolted from the table. I ran upstairs to my bedroom and locked the door, wishing I would never have to look at any of them ever again.

"If there were heartfelt words of compassion that were spoken to try and soothe my humiliation, I never heard them. I don't remember anything but the immense embarrassment of having my secret life exposed. Despite my parents' best efforts, the only immediate impact this exposure had on me was to make me even more determined to continue my covert consumption of food.

"This incident has earned a revered place in my family's history. Everyone knows about it and we all have our own opinions concerning it. We've never really discussed it, as if the event itself is the definitive feature and there's nothing more to say. Mostly, my family thinks it's funny, just another humorous anecdote. At family gatherings, if someone inadvertently mentions doughnuts, gazes will land on me. 'Knowing' smiles will come across faces and I will inevitably blush.

"No one in my family has ever bothered to ask if this event has had a lasting impact on me. If they had, I would tell them that it has made me a better parent than I ever dreamed I would be. It has taught me to speak to my son and to encourage him to speak to me. I have learned to respect his privacy, help him face his fears and instill in him a good sense of self that will carry him into the future. More than anything, it has taught me to strive to show compassion. Lastly, it's taught me to appreciate my son's love of doughnuts."

» «

Mitch is overweight because he eats, and because he is genetically predisposed to being overweight, and because his mother is morbidly obese. It's simply part of his makeup, and he will have to fight it every day for the rest of his life. Still, he has no idea how lucky he is to have a mother who is understanding and compassionate, who truly gets what he's going through and is savvy enough to leave him alone.

Lots of people won't think so, of course. Instead, they'll see a fat mother with a fat child and immediately break into condemnation mode. It takes a mighty tough person not to feel like a failure when the entire world is telling you that you are. But it is possible—which recalls Anamarie Regino.

You might know the story: Ana was the three-year-old, 120-pound girl in Albuquerque, New Mexico, who was taken from her parents because she was too fat. The story was splashed all over the airwaves; parents of overweight kids across the country were terrified that they might be next, that the state might barge in like the Gestapo and remove their child.

Ana was a medical anomaly. At eight months, she weighed thirty-eight pounds; at twelve months, she already had two rows of teeth, and her hair was thicker than a five-year-old's. She drank ten to twelve bottles a day and hungered for more. The endocrinologist told her mother, Adela Martinez-Regino, that Ana was just going to be big. At two, she couldn't walk. Her bones and muscles couldn't support her seventy-pound frame. A bone scan showed her to have the bones of a four- or five-year-old when she was a year old.

The doctors had no idea what was wrong. Some thought it might be Prader-Willi Syndrome, a rare chromosomal disturbance in which children can become so ravenous that parents literally have to bolt the refrigerator. Children with Prader-Willi tend to be obese, and usually speak, walk, and toilet-train later than most children. But Prader-Willi patients typically have feeding problems as infants, which Ana never did. Plus, they're usually short for their ages, whereas Ana was taller than most of her friends.

The doctors tried varying her diet: 1,200 calories, 1,000 calories, 900, 500. Adela did everything they told her to, even putting her daughter on an unimaginable daily regime of two vanilla-flavored Kindercal drinks at 250 calories a pop. Again, nothing worked, Ana was still fat—130 pounds at age three—and doctors put her in a hospital program. She lost weight there, but as soon as she returned home it crept back on. Soon Adela, then thirty-three, realized that the doctors were beginning to suspect her and her husband, Miguel, fifty-three, of sabotaging Ana, of feeding her solid food when she was only supposed to drink liquids. Of deliberately keeping her large. Of child abuse. (They even thought Ana was a victim of Munchausen's Syndrome by Proxy, a psychological disorder in which parents deliberately hurt their offspring to call attention to themselves.)

In August 2000, the Reginos were asked to bring Ana to the hospital for even more tests, and checked her into the pediatric unit. A few days later a social worker told the couple that Ana was going to be taken from them and placed in foster care. And that is exactly what happened.

After Ana was removed, the Reginos made the rounds of TV and print media. They met with Diane Sawyer, whom they liked, and Katie Couric, whom they did not like as much (although they keep a photo of her with them on the living room wall). They found a lawyer, Troy Prichard, who offered his services pro bono after reading about the case. They also attracted the attention of several fat activists, many of whom testified on their behalf.

Prichard found Adela and Miguel another pediatrician, Javier Aceves, who was born in Mexico and could speak to Ana and her parents in English and Spanish, which no one else could. He increased her diet to 1,000 calories a day, with solid food. Anamarie lost weight—ten pounds during her first two months in foster care. At one point she was losing so fast that Aceves increased her daily calories to 1,200. To curb her sleep apnea, she slept with an oxygen machine, which Adela had been told to do but, caseworkers said, didn't properly implement.

In October, a few days before a hearing in which the state would be asked to show why Anamarie should continue to be separated from her parents, Prichard reached an agreement with the Children, Youth and Families Department. The state maintained legal custody of Ana, but she would be allowed to return to her parents, which she did on November 10. The only downside was the caseworkers who spent hours in the family's home, monitoring their every move.

By January, Ana was losing weight; a psychiatrist evaluated Adela and found no evidence of psychological problems. The judge dismissed the charges of abuse and returned legal custody to the Reginos. He eventually dismissed the case entirely, and though the Reginos considered a civil suit, they never moved forward with it.

Javier Aceves acknowledged that taking her away from her family probably wasn't the right choice, but he said that he completely understood why it had seemed to be the only option. He believes that Anamarie has some unnamed, unidentified metabolic problem, and that, commingled with parents who expressed their love with food, caused her to gain weight.

Adela told the *New York Times Magazine* that she was comforted every time Aceves admitted that he didn't know what was wrong with Ana, "because all those other doctors thought they knew and they ended up blaming us."

» «

Ever since I'd heard about Anamarie Regino, I'd wanted to meet her and her family. Her story hadn't been in the papers for a few years, and I wondered where—and how—she was. Finally, a member of the

National Association to Advance Fat Acceptance (NAAFA) who had lobbied on her behalf gave me the family's number. I left many messages and after a few months Adela returned my calls.

She was friendly on the phone, if a little wary, which was understandable. The family had been bombarded with press, who descended on their little street like the National Guard. She told me I was welcome to interview her, but not when Ana was around. "You can meet her, but I don't want her to hear us talking, she'll understand," she says. In the past, "She didn't understand really why everybody was wanting to know her. She still doesn't, but she's catching on. She's still very afraid of people."

Fair enough.

I visit one afternoon in September 2003, hot as a skillet, every curl sucked out of my hair. The Regino house is small and somewhat downtrodden, in a mostly Mexican neighborhood. The place is decorated modestly, frugally. Photos of Anamarie line the walls, a palpable chart of her soaring weight over the years.

Adela brings home $614 every two weeks, after taxes, from her job as a counter-agent for Mesa Airlines. Her house payment is $725 a month; she has no credit card, and never eats out. Miguel, now fifty-five, a former painter in a cabinet shop with five children from a first marriage, went on disability for diabetes three years ago. He gets $723 a month. Ana gets $2,000 a month in social security because of her disability. "What's her disability?" I ask, settling on the couch.

"They don't know. She has an Unknown."

According to Sandra Solovay, a civil rights lawyer and author of *Tipping the Scales of Justice* (Prometheus Books, 2000), obesity is not automatically covered by disability law, but extreme fat is considered an impairment under the law. According to the Department of Justice, "It is generally accepted that morbid obesity, which is defined as body weight 100 percent over normal weight, is an impairment."

Adela, who is four foot eleven and round—plump, actually—is still angry about what happened to her daughter. She repeats the story I've read many times over, and listening to her talk I can't help but think of her as the victim of a terrible tragedy. I admit it: I had condemned her, too. How else does a child get so big if her parents aren't overfeeding her? People do it all the time. And I understand the state's concern: 120 pounds is big for a three-year-old. And yet the more I hear Adela talk, the more I believe her. Ana obviously has a medical condition.

"After all that went on, the doctors still don't know what's wrong with Ana," Adela says bitterly. "I'm accepting my daughter but I would still like to know." A few diet doctors have called wanting to help her out but only "so they could promote their stuff," Adela notes wryly.

Obesity doesn't run in her husband's family, though diabetes does. One of her uncles is heavy, and her mother once weighed 200 pounds, which she has since lost.

The doctors think Ana will menstruate early. Adela did, at age nine, when she was in the fourth grade. That's when she started gaining weight.

"But I was a normal baby. The most I've ever been was twenty pounds overweight. There's really not been that many people in our family that had weight as big as Ana until they were adults. Food has never really been a big issue in our family. We were always taught to share. I was fat and my sister was thin. I dealt with it when I was in school. It bothered me because I was overweight and I didn't get the guys, but I'm okay with how I am now. I wish I was skinnier, but I'm not going to diet."

Adela mistrusts everyone, and thinks everyone has ulterior motives. For example, she believes the state wanted her daughter for medical research. "I would see marks under her arms and I was like, 'What is going on?' They had her on a monitor at night, which was for SIDS [Sudden Infant Death Syndrome]. A SIDS monitor!" She has worked herself into a frenzy. "She had sleep apnea and they figured that if she stopped breathing this machine would go off, but this machine isn't good for children her age because they move too much. She was on a couple of other machines and no one could tell me why she was hooked up to them. Which makes me think they just wanted to use her and see what was happening with her."

"How's her weight today?" I ask.

"Fine," she says. "I don't make a big deal out of it. I used to when the state was involved. I would panic and think, 'Oh my God.'

"I was always taught not to fight about food or make food a big subject," she continues. "They think 'Hispanics, all their universe is around food.' It's not. I used to have candies around. She wouldn't go after them and to this day she doesn't."

Adela monitors what her daughter eats. Everything is measured and weighed both at home and at school. She swears Ana eats only 1,000 calories a day, that she doesn't swap food at school. I find it hard to believe. I couldn't even live on 1,000 calories. And every kid shares food at school. But Adela says no. "Ana's around people who know what she can eat and what she can't. I have always told Ana, 'Your body works differently. You're not any different than this person. You may be taller or bigger.' She's the tallest one in her class."

Not that they try to ostracize her or make her feel weird. "If they have a birthday party she's allowed to get a piece of cake just like anybody else." But Ana isn't like every other kid. "You know how kids go and grab? Not Ana, she'll ask you. She's very afraid of other people seeing her eat, too. I don't want to make it where she's embarrassed to eat."

That said, Ana has been known to sneak food—even apples. "I told her, 'I don't want you ever hiding anything from me,'" Adela says, grimacing at the memory. "'We don't hide food here. We share food. You don't have to be ashamed of eating anything and I don't care what it is—ice cream or an apple or banana.'"

Adela blames the state for Ana's fears around food. Often, when Ana was in the hospital, she would be served a meal that would be quickly removed. "She would get upset. You're taking away her food! Of course she got upset," Adela says. "She caught on to that so when they would feed her again she would eat quickly. That's when they tried to say she had Prader-Willi, that she didn't know when to stop. They thought she was harboring food because she ate so fast. They gave her that problem. She eats too fast because she's afraid of someone coming and taking her food."

Ana, who is now six, is afraid someone will take her food; Adela and Miguel worry that someone will take away their daughter. Every time the phone or doorbell rings they jump, three years after the fact.

Over the years Adela has overhauled her kitchen and learned about nutrition. She keeps fruits and vegetables around the house. If Adela wants something sweet—she's a Coke fiend—she'll take it to work and drink it there. "I've learned how to make tortillas the healthy way. We cook it with a little bit of oil and not as much fat. When I grew up and started learning to make tortillas I was making them with lard. Now I cook them with oil. You can't tell any difference.

"If parents were taught healthy ways I think they would change," she says. "I've learned a lot of stuff. Basic stuff like you look at the fat intake, look at the sugar. In the past, we were buying yogurt and I was buying the one that had more sugar. But I didn't know."

And they exercise—well, try to, anyway. They walk to school every day, and after school hit the park. Ana has gym and walks on the treadmill ten to fifteen minutes every day. "The physical therapist said even a minute would be okay, don't push her. *I'm* the overachiever. *I'm* the one wanting more. These therapists are like, 'No, as long as she's doing it that's all that matters.'"

Ana also goes to physical therapy. And speech therapy. And occupational therapy, where she's been learning how to brush her hair, put her clothes on, tie her shoes—things she has trouble with apparently because of her unnamed, undiagnosed disorder.

"What I like about when I take her to therapy is that they get her to work without her knowing that she's working," Adela says. "These people have gotten her further than the therapist before. Before, anytime I said, 'It's time to go to therapy' or we got in the car she would kick and scream. She didn't want to go. Now she gets excited about it. It's an independent therapy place with a variety of kids, not just fat ones. I think Ana is the one case of overweight there. They make it fun for her."

But on the whole, Ana does not like to move. In her ideal world, she would play with her beads, tool around on the computer, or paint. And she's into cheerleading. Adela, proud mama that she is, points to the pictures on the wall: Ana in cheerleading outfit; Ana in her class photo; Ana as an enormous three-year-old, her eyes hidden behind thick glasses, her features hidden beneath masses of flesh.

"Does she ever say, 'I want to be thin'?" I ask. "Does she ever say, 'I'm too fat'?"

"Never!" her mom says. "The only thing that bothers her is that she has always wanted a Barbie jacket, but they don't make them in her size."

As for weighing her, well, at one point the state bought them three scales for daily weigh-ins. That was disastrous. "At the doctor's office the first thing the doctors do is weigh you. She got on the scales and she would look at us to see what our reaction was. Then she could tell if it was good or bad. That was very hard. We looked like failures. Even if it's just a pound—that's a really big weight gain."

So they stopped weighing her, and Adela has forbidden the school from doing so. "That is none of their business," Adela says firmly. "It's between me and the doctor."

But the hypocrisy really gets her.

"Here in New Mexico they're trying to get kids to eat healthy. This is what Albuquerque school lunches consisted of: peanut butter and jelly sandwich, white bread, potato chips, an apple, and whole milk. How much sugar does jelly have? The white bread is not healthy. Potato chips! They're trying to get kids to eat healthy and they're giving the kids potato chips!"

She's on a roll now. "And they're cutting phys ed! They're cutting things that should be out there to help kids! Yeah, computers are great, but you also have to have that kid go to PE and cutting that program is not helping."

What's more—and this is a big problem for lower income families—eating healthy is expensive. "If you're going to get people to eat healthy, lower the prices. McDonald's is cheap. You can't eat a healthy meal for that price. That's why people go to the fast food. Groceries cost about $100 a week. I go to Sam's Club. Sam's doesn't have a lot of diet stuff. I like it because they have lean meat, but they don't have lean snacks. Their fruit is very reasonable but even there it is expensive. It's just not cheap to eat healthy and that is a big problem."

"No one ever came to us and said, 'What does Ana eat?' or followed us to see what Ana eats. No one ever did that."

"Okay," I say. "Tell me what she eats."

"In the morning she has an egg fried with Pam and then she has cereal with skim milk. She drinks skim milk. That's all she has been drinking. Her fruit and that's it. That is her breakfast. For lunch she gets a half of sandwich with wheat bread, cheese, and your ham or whatever. Then you get your vegetables if there are any vegetables and she gets yogurt and she gets her fruit. That is all she eats. She can have one snack which is fruit and yogurt and a vegetable. I try to get away from the starch stuff.

"For dinner we have a half-portion of meat. Then we have a potato or tortilla, whatever starch we have and our vegetable. Then her fruit. I've tried because I have learned if you eat more protein like the Atkins diet it's a lot better than starchy food."

She offers to let me look around the kitchen, and I do. Her place is small and cluttered and things are everywhere, but it's pretty much devoid of any unhealthy foods, at least on the surface.

"Would you like her to lose weight?" I ask when we return to the living room.

Adela shrugs. "I'm fine with the way she is. I would like her to be more mobile. I would like her to feel comfortable. The only reason that I considered weight as a problem is that it was holding her back from walking. She never learned how to crawl because she was so big. It was too much on her bones. Right now when she can't do something I say, 'You can't do it because you don't want to do it. You can do anything you want. There's nothing holding you back. If you want to go and do it as long as you put your mind to it you can do anything you want.' I've never told her, 'You're too big' or 'You're slow' or 'You're too huge.' It's hard sometimes because she says, 'I can't do it as fast as they can.' I go, 'How about you practice?'"

123

Adela's biggest project is a scrapbook for Ana, a record of everything that's happened "so that when she gets older she can understand what happened. Why we will never know, but at least I can tell her my version. This is what happened. This is how we handled it. This is what we did."

"What else could you have done?" I ask.

She doesn't miss a beat; clearly, she's thought about this. "Maybe insisted more. I was brought up that all these doctors had high education, they know better. But they don't. I used to wonder, 'Should I stay home with her? Should I have not gone back to work? Did I measure wrong? What could we have done differently?' You think, 'Wait a minute, did I not ask for the right help?' But I don't blame myself anymore. All I can think of is she is going to grow up to be normal weight and she can come and say, 'Look at what happened to me and look at what I went through.'"

Just as we are finishing up Anamarie shuffles in, huffing like a pack-a-day smoker. She wears glasses and her hair is shoulder length and thick; like most six-year-olds, she is missing two front teeth. She speaks Spanish-inflected English, and she's hard to understand.

Let me say this: Anamarie is *big*. There's no question about that: 180 pounds of flesh. She is also tall—four foot three—well above average for her age. She looks ten. She asks her mom if she can have a Diet Coke. Her mom says yes, and Anamarie shyly offers me one, too, which I happily accept. She is sweet. I can imagine her having no idea what happened to her, or why, and I only hope she grows up knowing that her parents loved and accepted her when the rest of the world didn't.

» «

Unconditional love is the ideal. It's what we're supposed to strive for in all of our relationships. But when it comes to weight, parents have to tread mighty carefully. You can't be too accepting—as some families know all too well.

Indeed, the Reginos aren't the only family who were taken to court for raising a fat child. In February 2001, an Indianapolis mother named Heather Andis pleaded guilty to child neglect in the case of her five-year-old son, Cory, whose weight had once reached 138 pounds.

But perhaps the most famous case took place in San Francisco, circa 1996, when Marlene Corrigan, the mother of a thirteen-year-old girl named Christina, came home to find her daughter lying dead on the couch. Her nude body was sheathed in a dirty sheet, with empty fast-food wrappers and feces strewn about. She had open bedsores. It took six people to lug her body out of the house. She weighed 680 pounds. According to a medical examiner, Christina died of heart failure due to morbid obesity. Her mother was charged with child abuse and endangerment, a felony, despite the fact that Christina never had a proper autopsy.

The case became a media frenzy. Sondra Solovay, the civil rights lawyer, says the case had nothing to do with Christina's weight but with her living situation and the condition of her body. "The crime scene included photographs of a pizza box just the way they would snap a shot of a used bullet casing in a shooting," writes Solovay. "Pictures were taken of the contents of the refrigerator and freezer and trash was removed from bags and spread out on the living room floor for the photographic purposes. The judge in the hearing concluded that there was evidence of guilt of a felony, saying, the mother was the food source, she had ultimate control over what was being provided to the child."

"Good," says fourteen-year-old, 250-pound Emily Williams when I tell her what happened to Marlene. "A thirteen-year-old weighed 680 pounds! When she was 200 pounds her mother should have made her do something and not let her just lie around."

"But Emily—your mom doesn't have control over you," I said. "If something happens to you because of your weight, is she at fault?"

"My mother could, like, get me liposuction before I killed myself," she insists. "Most fat people don't reach 680 pounds in their entire life. They stay at, like, 350. To weigh 680 at age thirteen, how much could this girl be eating?"

It's a valid question. How could a thirteen-year-old reach nearly 700 pounds without someone, somewhere, stepping in? More to the point, how does anyone reach 700 pounds?

The answer is simple: Genetics. Not willpower. Not a lack of moral fiber. Just the genetic roll of the dice.

Researchers at Rockefeller University in Manhattan found that genetics could account for up to 80 percent of weight. They found that a 10 percent weight loss triggered a 15 percent reduction in metabolism, and that the body defends against unnatural weight gain the same way, increasing the metabolic rate with a weight gain of 10 percent.

Louis Aronne, director of the Comprehensive Weight Control Program at New York–Presbyterian Hospital and president of the North American Association for the Study of Obesity, believes that obesity is controlled by a "powerful biological system of hormones, proteins, neurotransmitters and genes that regulate fat storage and body weight and tell the brain when, what and how much to eat. . . . Once people gain weight, then these biological mechanisms, which we're beginning to understand, develop to prevent people from losing weight. It's not someone fighting willpower. The body resists weight loss."

Whether Christina Corrigan's environment affected her metabolism or whether she had genetic and endocrine abnormalities (most likely she suffered from Prader-Willi) is something no one will ever know for sure. But Marlene Corrigan was a single mother who held down two jobs while also caring for her aging parents, who died a few months after Christina. Police interviews with the Corrigan family indicate that the family knew Christina had a problem but they were completely baffled by it. So, it seems, were doctors. Marlene had taken her daughter to nutritionists and pediatricians, but gave up after nothing helped. She said she hoped that Christina would decide on her own to stop eating so much. Unfortunately, Marlene told police, Christina demanded food and she usually gave in.

Marlene's sister, Sandy Bickers, said she had been so upset about Christina's weight that she had called child welfare officials some years back. A caseworker visited when Christina was seven and weighed 200 pounds. She said the house smelled of urine, but officials didn't do anything about the weight problem because they believed it was under control.

The principal at Christina's elementary school also claimed teachers were concerned about the girl's weight, but since she seemed so well adjusted they didn't think it was necessary to intervene. Eight months after Christina died, after a trial by judge, Marlene Corrigan was sentenced to probation and community service. Her charges were reduced to a misdemeanor (passive child endangerment) from a felony (child abuse).

Size activists—those who fight for the rights of the obese—maintain there was much more to the story than the mainstream press reported. According to Solovay, Marlene was always trying to get her daughter, who loved to read and swim and dreamed of being a marine biologist, to lose weight. Christina had seizures as a baby and the doctors put her on Phenobarbital, which depresses the central nervous system. Her weight was average at three months and then below average, and Marlene was told not to use whole milk in her bottle.

How did she get so fat? Dr. Diane Budd, an endocrinologist at the University of California, San Francisco, who testified in Marlene's defense, believes that that very first diet may have altered her metabolic rate, causing her to gain weight. The weight gain was too fast to be explained by mere overeating. "By age three Christina weighed as much as an average eight-and-a-half-year-old. At five, after two more years of dieting, she weighed as much as a thirteen-year-old. At seven, she was over 180," Solovay writes.

Doctors found nothing out of the ordinary, although they never photographed her brain or sent her to a geneticist. Christina was put on a diet and given ceramic food to teach portions. She was weighed every two weeks, in a public area with nurses, staff, and other patients milling about. Still, she gained weight.

Everyone was frustrated: Marlene, Christina, the doctors. Mother and daughter went on diets together, they exercised, but still Christina gained weight.

When Christina was thirteen, she decided to quit junior high. In part her decision was about psychological self-preservation: Her peers abused her. But it was also about physical preservation. Her high school was at the top of a long hill, and she could no longer make the trek.

Like any mother, Marlene was concerned. She called the school and explained that her daughter was having difficulty getting around. They told her there was nothing they could do because obesity was not a disability.

Eventually Marlene decided to homeschool Christina, but was told that she couldn't do it unless she was certified. She could ill afford to hire a teacher, so she bought some books for her daughter and had her write book reports. The school never followed up.

After Christina died Marlene requested an internal autopsy, but she never got one. The doctor said he never received a request. Instead, he performed a ten-minute external autopsy and concluded that Christina died of heart failure. He was unaware of her history of seizures.

Marlene Corrigan was found guilty of a misdemeanor and sentenced to community service, counseling, and probation. I tried to contact her, but her lawyer told me she had died of cancer. She was forty-one years old.

» «

Is raising an obese child a form of abuse? Is accepting an obese child the way she is and not forcing her to lose weight a criminal offense? Is a parent liable if he doesn't insist his kid start a drastic diet or undergo gastric bypass surgery? Conversely, what if the child has surgery and dies on the table? If a child is fat, what does that say about you, the parent? If the Reginos were a wealthy, white, professional family, would their daughter have been taken away? (It's a good question, especially when you consider that there has not been one documented case of an anorexic kid being removed from her family.)

And what if you're simply not aware that your child is fat?

It's possible. Alison Jeffery, a member of the research team at the Peninsula Medical School in Plymouth, England, questioned 300 seven-year-old children and their parents about their perceptions of body size. One third of mothers and half of fathers who were either overweight or obese rated themselves as "about right." When the child was overweight but not obese, only a quarter of the parents knew it. But when the youngsters were obese, 40 percent of parents were not concerned about their child's weight. Most likely it's because parents are so used to seeing overweight youngsters that they don't realize when their own children are obese. Should that be considered a crime?

Sondra Solovay says no.

Fat, and the rights of those who battle it, is a subject she's passionate about. She's got her own food craziness, having grown up in a weight-obsessed household. "Everyone in my family has had something with their weight or had something to say about someone else's weight," she admits. "I'd spent my entire youth dieting—there was no one who could bug me more than I could bug myself. When I was in the eighth grade I was wearing Levis that were a thirty-three-inch waist—that's big if you're a teenager. I did all of the crazy diets."

Solovay, thirty-four, went to Brown University, devoted a lot of energy to women's causes, and was very active politically. At one point, an acquaintance asked her if she would be willing to talk publicly about her eating disorder.

Solovay has a big hearty laugh, which she uses often. "She assumed I had one because I was fat! I told her, 'I can't do that, because I don't have an eating disorder.' I'm a vegetarian and have been one since I was eleven. People can't believe it. They have such stereotypes. Once, I edited a magazine for fat women and we got a call from a Los Angeles college—would we like to come have a debate, the fat people versus the vegetarians? I was like, 'What side do you want me to be on? I'm fat and a vegetarian!' People can't believe that I'm a vegetarian."

But Brown was a cocoon; the rest of the world was not so amenable. A few years ago she was flying back from L.A., having won a big award from NAAFA. She got on Southwest Airlines—this was before it instituted its two-seats-for-the-price-of-one-fat-person policy.

"I was told I'd have to buy another seat but that 'We don't have another seat, so you can't go on this flight,'" she recalls, her laugh gone. "I was shocked, and my mother, who is also an attorney but not an activist, advocated for me. I got on the plane. Today I don't think I would be able to since they reinvigorated that policy."

Solovay thinks parents need to deal with their own issues—although she acknowledges that this is much easier said than done. "As a parent you're in quite a quandary," she says. "You side with society and tell your kid there's something wrong with him and subject the kid to a life of poking and prodding, but you're probably not providing the kid with a great life.

"I certainly think after Marlene took Christina to the doctor a hundred times and no one knew what was going on—like Adela Regino—she said, 'I'm going to do the best I can,'" she says.

Which brings me back to the original question. Can parents be sued for having an obese child? Should they be?

In her book, Solovay cites the case of one family, pseudonymously called the Smullers. The father worked out of town and only spent weekends with his family. When he was around he constantly harangued his son, Zack, about his weight.

When the couple divorced, both wanted custody. The father's lawyer said that Mrs. Smuller was an unfit mother because her son was fat.

In this instance, both parents were thin, but had one been heavy, Solovay says, the judge could have ruled against her, since "she was a bad role model because of her own weight." (The Smullers ultimately settled out of court.)

"Even in cases where the child is without the added risk of a specific condition worsened by weight, the courts have shown a willingness to consider the weight of the child when making custody and guardianship decisions," Solovay writes. "Whether the court will make a negative custody determination based on the child's weight depends on the particular state's laws or case law, and on the individual judge's opinions and prejudices."

Another case is *Fillingim v. Fillingim*, which took place in 1980 in Montgomery, Alabama. The Fillingims' five-year-old son, Jimmy, had a history of "infrequent but severe grand mal seizures," says Solovay. The parents divorced, and a custody battle ensued. The mother, Diane, felt that her ex-husband, who had moved, lived too far away from a hospital should Jimmy need help. Medical experts even testified on behalf of the mother, saying that they had never seen the father.

Despite this, the judge increased the father's visitation rights, including overnight stays. He then held Mrs. Fillingim in contempt of court for refusing to allow the father visitation.

Ostensibly, the trial was about visitation. But since Jimmy weighed more than he should have, the judge ordered Mrs. Fillingim to put her son on a weight-reduction program. She was also ordered to report his weight to the court each month.

She appealed, and argued that the lower court had overstepped its bounds with the weight loss and the reporting requirements. The Alabama Court of Civil Appeals disagreed.

In February of 1980, Jimmy was four feet tall and weighed seventy-five pounds. He gained twenty-five pounds over the next seven months. His mother took him to doctors but none put him on a diet. Jimmy's pediatrician had been taking note of his weight, but never discussed it with his mother.

Mrs. Fillingim reduced the size of her son's meals and "eliminated some objectionable foods therefrom," Solovay writes. But the court said that she hadn't put him on a sufficient diet. This enrages Solovay. "If not the reduction of food intake and the elimination of 'objectionable' foods, then what does a diet entail? More important, what authority does the court have to determine that Ms. Fillingim's program is not a sufficient diet? And why is the court prescribing a diet for a five-year-old boy when the two physicians in charge of the boy's care chose not to?"

Although the appeals court basically supported the lower court's decision, it did rule significantly on two counts. "First, it curtailed the judge's power, indicating it might be unlawful for him to prescribe 'any medication, diet, exercise, or the type of weight program to be undertaken.' The court was not distressed that the lower court judge had dismissed the diet Ms. Fillingim put her child on, despite the fact that this would most likely have been precisely the diet a sensible doctor would have prescribed (reduced portions and elimination of certain foods)," Solovay writes. Nor was the court troubled by the judge's requirement that the child lose weight without making any attempt to ascertain the cause of the weight gain—was it normal? Was it due to his seizure medication? Was it a symptom of a hidden metabolic disorder? Was it a psychological reaction to the stress of divorce and his father's new family? Similarly, the court did not require the judge to check with a medical professional to be certain weight loss was even appropriate and safe for a five-year-old. Today, responsible endocrinologists and nutritionists would not put the child on any diet as they have come to realize the particular dangers of dieting for young children. Even then a doctor would likely have vetoed the judge's order, opting to let the child "grow into" his weight. Instead, the appeals court states, "The judge had a discretion to exercise in Jimmy's best interest, and he did so."

"Even when children and their parents are united in agreement that forced diets and commitment to an inpatient diet program are inappropriate, the family is still nearly powerless in the face of a judge who disagrees," Solovay writes. "But parents and children do not always agree on what's in the child's best interest. Children who are alone in their desire not to be forced into a diet have even less power."

Which leads me to wonder: What about all the anorexic children out there? Are their parents ever sued for neglect? Are there custody battles over depressed children, or autistic, or those with leukemia? Are parents blamed if their child is in a wheelchair or has seizures?

Unlikely. "If she had seizures, or was in a wheelchair, people would have seen the mother as almost a martyr," Judy Freespirit, a NAAFA spokesperson, commented in *Salon* on the Corrigan case. "But with a child who is fat, not only would she have to deal with this disabled child, but with the disapproval of everyone around her and the blame that somehow she should have stopped her daughter from eating."

Although in theory I agree with Solovay and Freespirit, in truth I'm not quite sure where I fall on this scale. Clearly, Christina Corrigan and Anamarie Regino are unique cases; it's simply not normal—and I use the term comparatively, based on the average weights of most American children—for a six-year-old child to weigh 180 pounds, let alone 680. But then, these girls *weren't* the average people; this *was* normal for them. That's the way their bodies were designed.

"I told the judge the parents are not responsible for how the child's body turns out," says Joanna Ikeda, codirector of the University of California, Berkeley's, Center for Weight and Health, who spoke on behalf of the Regino family. "After Christina died, a registered dietitian was quoted in the *San Francisco Chronicle* as saying that parents of fat kids should be put in jail for child neglect. I couldn't believe that someone who was trained and knows about all of the factors and the development for obesity and how much we don't know would actually say that. I suppose if parents deliberately made the decision to deliberately foster obesity in their child, yes, but what kind of bizarre parent is that?

"One thing's for sure, she's never going to be skinny," she continues. "But maybe if she practices safe sex and wears a seat belt she'll be okay. If she gets diabetes, then you treat the diabetes or whatever she comes down with. You're assuming there's something one can do; there are limits to even medical science."

In a statement about the case, Ellyn Satter said: "The issue of childhood obesity is complex, and the ability of clinicians, let alone the legal profession, to sort out the complexity is rare. Was Anamarie too fat? She looks fat, but you can't tell by just looking, or even by comparing her weight with cutoff points on a weight-for-height or body mass index chart. You can only tell by examining weight records from birth. Has Anamarie been consistently fat from the time she was a baby? If so, her fatness is natural or normal for her. Contrary to the popular assumption that we should all come from the same size-and-shape cookie cutter, some children are normally fat.

"If, on the other hand, Anamarie's weight has diverged upward on the growth charts as she has gotten older, we have to ask ourselves why. It is normal for children to eat normally, grow consistently and achieve their constitutional endowment for size and shape. If they don't, something is seriously wrong. It takes a lot to make a child gain too much weight. To locate the source of the disruptions requires a careful and detailed evaluation of past and present medical, social, developmental and environmental issues.

"Children don't just automatically get fatter than nature intended them to be—there are reasons. A child may have been temperamentally difficult, hard to reach and hard to discipline so parents have used food to comfort, connect or subdue. Parents may have been frightened by a child's early health problems and have overfed because of anxiety about the child's survival. But overfeeding is not common. To overfeed, parents have to consistently feed beyond the child's signs of fullness, meal after meal, day after day. Children compensate—they make up for parents' errors in feeding by not getting hungry as quickly or by eating less the next time.

"In my clinical practice, I have found that once the source of the problem is identified, most parents can follow a reasonable course of action. A weight-reduction diet is not reasonable. Not feeding a child enough is policing, not parenting. Instead, parents can optimize: provide regular meals and snacks, limit the child's in-between grazing for food, give opportunities to be active, and parent in such a way that the child feels safe. Given optimum parenting, children can be allowed to grow up to get the body that is right for them. If they are fat, so be it.

"Some parents need ongoing support or psychotherapy to get to the point where they can act in the best interest of the child.

Others demonstrate that they are incapable, even with help. Only when the family is truly incapable of providing for the child can removal from the home be legitimately considered."

Ongoing support and psychotherapy are good things. But I take it a step further. I think parents need to examine their own issues about food. Before bothering their kids, parents should call attention to their own eating habits. After all, how do we help our kids, if not by fixing the addictions in us? Fixing our addictions to Diet Coke, to nagging, to running, to eBay. Before we try to fix our children, we'd better worry about ourselves.

Danielle Webber is thirteen years **old**, four foot eleven, and weighs 137 pounds, down from 145. In the summer of 2003 she spent two weeks at the Pritikin Resort and Spa, in Aventura, Florida, with her grandfather, who has been going there for years to help with his blood pressure, cholesterol, and weight. Pritikin runs family programs every summer to teach kids the benefits of their ways. Danielle says she learned a lot, and Pritikin really helped her figure out how to eat, since she never knows what kind of diet her family will be on at a given time.

"When I was little my mom used to make us lasagna and pasta and she used to eat and so would my dad. But then all of a sudden, they started doing all these hard-core diets. And everything changed. I'd come home from school and my mom would say, 'I was walking in a store and they had a great thing that looked like a great diet.' And then that would be the new diet for the week," says Danielle, who lives in Miami. "We've been on a protein diet, Sugar Busters, the South Beach Diet as a family. Sometimes I'll be sarcastic and say, 'So, Mom, what diet are we on now?'"

Although Danielle is far from obese, her weight has been a family battle. Both of her parents—who also have slight weight problems—have given her a hard time about her size, which is why they sent her to Pritikin. "Before, my mom and my dad were like, 'You need to get on the treadmill and give me twenty minutes a day.' I don't like it when my parents do that. So one day I started yelling, 'It's my body and I will do what I want with it! You raised me well and I know how to exercise! If I want to exercise I can, and leave me alone with the food!' My mom said, 'Okay, but I won't leave you totally alone.'"

She's also not shy about speaking up to her dad. "He can yell at me all he wants but I know he's not perfect. So if he says, 'Oh my gosh, Danielle, don't eat that because you're overweight,' I just get so mad and I'll say, 'You're not Mister Perfect, either.' My mom will look at me and say, 'Good job!' because you can't criticize somebody if you're not perfect yourself."

» «

Tammy Cohen, being Tammy, wasn't content to just have KIC meetings. And it was getting difficult: a lot of the parents couldn't make them. So she decided it was time to implement phase two of her program, the exercise component, with the kids.

Seventeen kids showed up to the pilot. The deal—the way Tammy sold it to them—was to weigh them first, in the beginning, and then to tell them how much muscle they have. Not weight, but muscle.

"They don't know their weight or their BMI," she says. "We're teaching them to be healthy, it's not about weight. We want them to jump around."

So the kids do it. They play basketball and hockey and do yoga. They climb a wall and kickbox. They run around and whoop it up. They look . . . *happy*.

No, Tammy's not perfect, but she has a learning curve, she takes responsibility for her own behavior, and she's trying to help her child. She has learned the important lessons: To focus on yourself in addition to worrying about your offspring. To provide structure. To model the behavior you want your kid to exhibit. Sometimes she slips, and sometimes she forgets, and sometimes she wants to run for the hills. But she is trying. That's about all we can ask of anyone.

4

the myths of
willpower and
control

h ere was the real problem with fat camp: It ended. Oh, I lost
weight—it's impossible not to with an enforced program—
but once you return to the real world, to the White Castles and
Whitman Samplers, to the macaroni and cheese and McDonald's,
to the refrigerator and school lunch and neighborhood delis, you're
going to encounter a lot of temptation. It takes a lot of inner
strength to withstand it, which most adolescents simply don't have.
No place can change a lifetime of learned habits in two months.

The first year, I lost fifteen pounds in nine weeks. (Not quite
what I'd hoped, alas; the plan was to get *underweight* so I'd have ten
pounds to play with.) When I returned home for my senior year of
high school, I was lean and muscular and strong. My parents didn't
recognize me when I stepped off the plane. My grandmother saw
me and cried, "Hello, skinny!" Friends suggested I get mono more
often. I never felt so omnipotent and proud.

The euphoria lasted about three days. After everyone got over
their initial shock, things drifted back to normal. Though I may
have been a few pounds lighter, I didn't get the lead in the school
play; guys didn't pummel my door for dates; and my popularity
didn't automatically skyrocket. It was an interesting lesson, one I

still grapple with today. When something goes wrong my first instinct is to blame it on my weight, even though I'm in fairly good
condition. (So many women I know do the same thing—and, conversely, they feel that things are okay as long as the scale reads a certain number.) But it makes sense. It's a lot easier to swallow, being
rejected for what I look like than for who I am. It's a lot nicer to
think a man doesn't want me because I'm not a size 2 than because
he thinks I'm boring. Or antagonistic. Or unappealing. Or just not
his type.

Life as a thin person wasn't all it was cracked up to be. Physically,
I felt great, but I was terrified of eating, of blowing up like an elephant. Afraid that I'd have to admit failure and return to camp.

On the other hand, I would have loved to return to Camp
Colang—especially having maintained my weight—but I couldn't afford it and my parents thought it was ridiculous to spend money
when I would obviously be the smallest one there. But I missed the
camp environment; it was so safe, so easy. Someone else regulated
my meals, someone else told me what I could and couldn't eat, someone else made my choices. All I had to do was show up and sweat.
The fat farm sheltered me in a low-calorie womb that I was reluctant
to emerge from, and I found it liberating—ironic, I know, since
camp was constricting instead of freeing. Yet I honestly believed
that camp provided me with the chance to take a summer off from
thinking about food. (And what did I think about instead, you ask?
Oh, you know—my biceps, my pecs, how many inches I'd lost.) But,
as I later learned, I was wrong. The camp didn't liberate me from my
weight problem, it didn't liberate me from my obsession with food.
If anything, it heightened it. I grew to depend on these places, I
grew addicted to them like a bulimic grows addicted to laxatives. I
used camp as an escape. It was a safe refuge, a haven, for people who
couldn't cope in the real world. Oh, sure, on the surface it seemed as
if there were a higher purpose for my being there—to lose weight!—
but basically the fat farm was a place where I could hide.

After that first summer, I didn't know how to eat in the real
world. I was afraid to put anything into my mouth but still couldn't

fathom deprivation, so I devised a plan, a way to indulge myself but not feel restricted. I separated my life into two neat categories: food days and nonfood days. The latter were controlled with a surgeon's painstaking precision; the former, with the carefree mania of an addict.

The routine was always pretty simple. For three days I would diet religiously, eat 1,200 calories, and exercise with a vengeance. On the fourth day, the food day, I would wake up knowing that I wouldn't hold back, that I would suck on chocolate-covered cherries and fruit-flavored jellybeans and sponge cake as soft as cotton. I would drench pancakes in maple syrup, ice cream in butterscotch fudge. I would smother salads in blue cheese, potatoes in melted butter. My food days were minivacations, respites from the monotony of everyday life. Perhaps I felt I deserved them, that someone, somewhere, owed them to me. My most consistent relationship has been with food; I viewed these days as old friends I both treasured and despised. They were the only days I looked forward to.

Nonfood days, on the other hand, were the calm after the storm. On these days I coped, physically, with the aftermath of the previous day's damage, my body trying to heal itself from the destruction suffered at my own hands. I regulated my food intake with near-anorexic precision. Often I was hungry, daydreaming about blueberry muffins and peanut butter cookies and chocolate mousse, but I didn't eat them—that was strictly reserved for food days.

Not surprisingly, on nonfood days, while the acid in my stomach gurgled and the nausea slowly receded, I always ate by myself: a salad at Burger King, a Lean Cuisine at the kitchen table. I usually felt so sick from overeating I didn't even want to leave my bed, let alone the house. My stomach was too big, my face too bloated, my eyes so swollen I could hardly see. If I did go out that night, I couldn't—wouldn't—eat a meal unless I knew the exact caloric content (220 in a baked potato without sour cream; 150 per ounce of turkey). It really didn't bother me to just sit there, a cup of herbal tea in hand, while my companions' forks attacked their chicken a la king or fettuccine. It wasn't pleasure I derived from watching them eat. It's simply the way it was. But empty plates tend to unnerve people. Most people, I've discovered, don't like to indulge unless someone else joins in the fun.

Ironically, on the nonfood days, which unfortunately came too often, I longed to be with other people, hungered violently for a man, a woman, anyone to connect with. Maybe that's why I stuffed myself. Yet I never had a steady relationship: Relationships required too many explanations. I didn't want to worry about adjusting my food schedule to someone else's, didn't want to think about my body in relation to another's. I remember lying with a boyfriend—I must have been twenty-three—his arms wrapped around my waist, his hands stroking my stomach, my thighs. He held me, kissed me: the safest place in the world. And all I could think was: *I'm so fat.*

Besides, what if, God forbid, someone had the nerve to want to see me two, three, four days in a row? Right about then the panic would set in, a deep pit of fear that welled up in my stomach. How was I supposed to eat the way I wanted to when someone else wanted to go out for food, drinks—or worse—cook me a meal? Then the lying would kick in: *I always eat like a bird; I'm lactose intolerant, a vegetarian; I had a late lunch.* Anything so I wouldn't have to eat.

» «

One of my counselors from Colang had recommended Kingsmont, a weight-loss camp in West Stockbridge, Massachusetts (there's a lot of cross-pollination in the fat farm world), and it sounded great, a real mom and pop shop. The owner, or at least the adopted mascot, was a gentle old man called Doc whom all the kids adored. It seemed like a really loving place and it was near Tanglewood, so they had cultural field trips rather than mere shopping expeditions. And it was politically correct. Instead of Color War, for example, they had Color Games. Sounded perfect for me. So the summer before my freshman year of college I took a job as a counselor in training and got even more screwed up about food.

Kingsmont, I believe, encouraged more obsessive behavior than Colang. Or maybe it's just that I wasn't used to being a counselor and hadn't known how disturbed they could be. At night we would go to a diner on the Taconic Parkway and gorge; then we'd hit Price Chopper and fill our bags with jellybeans and chocolate-covered peanuts. On days off we would pig out and then amuse each other with consumption tales.

Kingsmont had a back room attached to the main dining hall. After meals the counselors would chow down on leftover pizza, macaroni, pudding—whatever remained. It wasn't as if we were hungry—it's just that the food was there, so why not eat it? The campers would lurk outside, bleating like goats, begging for handouts—they knew what was going on inside, even though we told them it was a "room of our own" for some peace of mind. But there's no mistaking the sound of a fork scraping the bottom of a bowl for the sound of one hand clapping. One girl, Angie, gained fifteen pounds that summer. Another counselor told me she gained and lost as much as eight pounds in one week because she was so bulimic. That back room only fueled her illness.

I left camp that summer a pound heavier than when I arrived, and with a pretty major bingeing problem.

By the time I finished my first semester of college I was twenty-six pounds heavier than when it began—heavier, even, than the first time I went to fat camp. My wardrobe options diminished. I alternated between a black sweat suit and a buttonless, zipperless frock that slipped over my head. But my oversized clothes didn't fool anybody, least of all me. My thighs still rubbed together, my breasts spilled out of my bra, my stomach bulged over my underwear. I was sure the first thing people thought when they saw me was, "How did she get so fat?" And I was.

I attended a small liberal arts college in Ithaca, New York, and studied Communications and Theater. My goal was to become the next Barbara Walters. "You'll be great as long as you're thin," my grandmother said. "Those women are all skinny."

At first, being away from home felt like someone had finally pulled a bath plug from my chest. I no longer felt choked, like my every move was being watched and graded. I didn't miss my family at all. I know my sister felt similarly when she went to Stanford, as if she could breathe for the first time in her life. She stayed there after graduation, got an MBA and a husband. Her panacea involved physical distance; mine involved the latest baked goods by Drakes.

But as the semester progressed my feelings of liberation dwindled. I didn't want to be back in Boston, but I didn't want to be at school, either. What I wanted to do—had fantasized about doing after graduating from high school—was take time off, float around the world, figure out why I was at school in the first place. But my parents, who were footing the bill, refused. "They all go straight to college," my mother said, invoking the mythical "them" into her logic. I still don't know who, or where, "they" were (David Letterman once claimed that "they" were the Van Pattens: Dick, Joyce, Vince, et al.), and whenever I asked she'd say, "Oh, you know exactly who I mean. People. The world. Them."

The longer I stayed at school the lonelier I became. The other kids—*them*—mingled happily, as if they were privy to some secret I wasn't. I wandered the hallways, the Student Union, looking for allies, but I couldn't find anyone. I'd hoped my roommate might be that person, that we'd have the kind of collegial bonding experience you see in movies, but it was clear from day one that would not be our fate. Amy was a bottle blonde who wept as soon as her mother, who had spent hours arranging her daughter's belongings, finally left. I didn't know what to do—ideally, move to a new room—but I sat down on Amy's Laura Ashley bedspread, put my arm around her shoulder, and told her it was natural to be homesick, that everything would be okay, that we were lucky to have each other, blah, blah, blah. I couldn't relate at all; when my folks finally left I lit a cigarette. I let her put on an Air Supply tape and started unpacking my own stuff. She was thrilled with the scale I brought, which I kept right on the floor by my bed, exactly eight inches away from the wall.

I suppose I did normal things at school—hung out, went to parties, had meaningless encounters with members of the opposite sex—but I always felt a fraud, and I was terribly, terminally lonely. I smoked pot and drank, but neither one was my drug of choice. Usually I consumed so much sugar I didn't need anything else, and no one knew the difference, anyway. With my slitted, swollen eyes and puffy cheeks, I always looked stoned.

It was during this period that I metamorphosed into Queen of the Deadheads. (Lest you aren't acquainted with hippie culture, the incense-waving followers of the Grateful Dead were dubbed "Deadheads," and I was one.) I truly believed that those earthy, unshaven granola-eaters were concerned with inner cores, souls. I thought they would accept me for who I was, not what I looked like, and I found that extraordinarily appealing. I decided to become the best damn hippie this side of Woodstock, and I embraced my new vocation with fervor and determination. I wore wraparound skirts. I tossed my razors in the garbage. (Once, at home for a few days, my mother told me I had to shave my legs. "Okay," I said. "But you do it for me." So we trooped into the backyard and sat on the picnic table and she shaved my legs in the sun.) I acquired the requisite collegiate Deadhead drawl—elongated vowels, lazy speech patterns, lots of *man*s and *dude*s—and grew passionate about Spring Tour. In retrospect, I should have been able to see through the facade, should have been tipped off by the Deadhead boys who lured you back to their room with talk of crystals and karma and the plight of being a sensitive male in an insensitive world, and then did everything in their power to get you into bed. "It's completely natural," they'd say, and, not wanting to be thought uncool or unnatural, you'd give in. And then, of course, they'd never call. They usually liked girls who shaved. Secretly I liked the jocks better, anyway. They, at least, made no pretenses about what they wanted, and I was on a quest for honesty, purity, "realness, man."

How I longed to be easygoing and free and uncomplicated. But I was a lousy Deadhead. I dressed the part and loved the music (and the shopping), but I had too much manic energy to really perfect it. Peace and love notwithstanding, I was the only hippie—hippie-crite, hippo-crite—I knew who carried around a bottle of lo-cal

Zesty Italian salad dressing in her oversized Guatemalan sack, which I'd acquired at a Grateful Dead show in Alpine Valley, Wisconsin, for $20 and a beer. I favored TV dinners over organic tofu; I was a jelly bean freak. And, of course, there was always the Electric Kool-Aid Diet Coke Test.

I'd been doing it for years, usually only when I ordered soda from a fountain. Having worked at McDonald's, I knew that the counter help sometimes erred and placed the cup beneath the Coke nozzle instead of Diet Coke. In my twisted, warped mind I sometimes believed they were deliberately trying to sabotage my diet.

"Taste this," I'd say, proffering my drink to whomever I was with. "Doesn't it taste sweet?" If no one was with me, I'd ask the counterperson, "Are you sure this is diet? I'm diabetic, you know, and I have to watch my sugar." (A lie.)

Invariably it was diet—the aftertaste gave it away—but on occasion there was some discrepancy (fountain is sweeter than canned, which is fizzier than bottled). No problem: I'd simply exchange the drink and watch to make sure they pressed the diet button.

Still, I tried to be a Deadhead. I decorated my bedroom with pictures of suns and moons and stars and the Queen of Swords, and I tacked a photograph of Jerry Garcia circa 1968 over my bed. I'd even student-directed a documentary entitled, *Dinner with the Dead*.

But I was miserable, still miserable. Always bingeing and starving, bingeing and starving. My friends tripped on acid. I OD'd on sugar. I spent Christmas vacation of my freshman year in Miami at a Weight Watchers camp for adults. It cost me $2,000. I lost seven pounds, which I gained back as soon as I returned to school.

And so in 1986 I went back to Colang, this time as a Collegiate. I weighed 147—twenty-five pounds heavier than the last time I had been there. It was mortifying.

"What happened to you?" people cried. "You were so thin when we last saw you!" Were they glad? Possibly. I was old now—eighteen—no longer a cute sixteen-year-old. The campers and counselors who knew me two years earlier were shocked that I'd gotten so big. Of course, there were kids much, much heavier than me—but still, I was a failure.

» «

Only recently have I begun to comprehend what a food problem—no matter what form it takes, no matter how much you weigh—does to the people in your life. (And I call it a food problem because I never really had an eating disorder. Americans form to fit labels—everyone's a Recovering Something—but I never fell into any one category. What was I? A normal-weight person with an anorexic mentality? A wannabe bulimic? Indeed, I'd mastered the binge; I just couldn't perfect the purge.) It tests them, pressures them, alienates them, really. People who can deal with it are in; those who can't are discarded like week-old pastry. A food and weight problem infects a relationship in subtle, insidious ways, as any addiction does. My good friends—those who *lived* with it—knew enough to ask before we made plans, "Is this a food day?" They knew that would determine how we'd spend our evening, whether we'd be dining out or simply watching a film.

Only recently have I understood my friend's frustrations, although for years they'd been trying to express them.

An ex-boyfriend, Ron, wrote a "fictional" story about a couple that fought bitterly, primarily because she refused to eat with him. He believed she used food as a way of withholding love. He thought she cared more about food than about him. In retrospect, he was probably right.

Tom, a potential lover, wanted to take me to dinner. "I can't go," I said simply. I waited for the anger, the incredulous stares, but Tom was in love with me and had all the patience in the world. Inevitably, though, he tired of eating alone. "Would you ever consider changing for anyone?" he asked. I was dumbfounded by this question. It had never crossed my mind.

Another boyfriend, Sam, would flit about my kitchen, a male Julia Child. Sam turned music up loud, filled my refrigerator with all sorts of food (he also loved to wear my dresses, but that's another story). One night he decided, on a whim, to invite friends for dinner; it was the first time, ever, I had done this. Sam whipped up a feast of garlic bread, noodles, and crepes. It was a beautiful creation, but there was a catch. I adored having him with me—he breathed life into my home—but even for him I would not, could not, eat. It just wasn't a food day. During dinner I jabbed at a dry, leafy salad, but I wouldn't sample anything else. Sam looked at me like a wounded puppy. "Why won't you eat my food?" he asked, scraping tomato sauce from a pan. I didn't feel close enough, comfortable enough, to explain it, so I mumbled some excuse about PMS. I would rather he think me rude than crazy.

Besides his cooking, Sam had one other flaw. He smoked too much pot, which I hated. He knew I felt this way, and so he snuck behind bushes when he wanted to get high. But I always knew. His eyes were rimmed with red and his face turned blank and everything about him became cloudy. Extremist that I am, I saw this as a symbol of what was wrong between us, a sign that clearly we had nothing in common. I took it as a personal affront, too, because he knew I hated it and yet he wouldn't stop. "If you know it bothers me," I finally demanded, "Why do you do it?"

Sam skipped a beat, and then said, "If you know how much I hate that you won't eat my food, that you eat candy behind my back, why won't you stop?"

And suddenly it hit me that we did have something in common: We were both addicts.

Sam is no longer in my life, but because of him I finally understand just how intimate an activity eating can be—an association that normally begins in the family. My apartment was never so alive as when a pot of soup was simmering on the stove, brownies baking in the oven. Because of Sam I learned to see food—the sharing of it, the preparation of it, the peculiar food-related decisions we make— as something almost mystical, a spiritual bond that connects people. Nothing seems as intimate as when a friend or lover pokes his fork into my plate or feeds me mouthfuls of chocolate cake. Of course, this awareness only intensifies my pain, my anger, because now I'm aware of all I've missed.

About twelve years ago I spent a week with friends in Chicago. For seven days we were a community, a family, cooking and eating together. Before one meal my friend Ilana asked me to sauté onions, dice carrots. I joked with her, making light of my ignorance, but I really had no idea what to do. Ilana found it endearing, but I was mortified.

I shouldn't have been, though. The truth is, I never had a need to learn about food. When I prepared a salad for myself, it didn't matter if the lettuce leaves were properly shredded, if the tomatoes were sliced to perfection. I just tossed everything in and ate. For someone so consumed with food, I had the palate of a pauper. I knew nothing about food: cooking it, preparing it, sampling it. I could wax poetic about the virtues of Tastykakes, could compare Healthy Choice to Lean Cuisine, but I couldn't talk knowledgeably about croque monsieurs or the different types of pasta.

And I was awkward, so awkward, at restaurants, dinner parties, business lunches, because I just wasn't used to them. When I was a child my mother taught me the significance of each fork, each glass, when to use which spoon, but as I grew older and more neurotic the need to know disappeared, replaced by cardboard containers and plastic forks. To this day, I feel as if I've been in a coma for the past twenty years and have had to slowly relearn how society functions.

» «

Food days and nonfood days still existed, of course, even in Chicago. Every third day I joined in for glasses of wine, crackers, and cheese, but on the other days I feasted on yogurt and fat-free apricot bars. (I was very thin at this point.) Ilana looked at me oddly, more sad than annoyed, but she'd known me long enough to know that's simply the way it was.

This doesn't mean she always understood. One Christmas I went to Mexico with her and her parents, who had lost, between them, over a hundred pounds. They understood—lauded, in fact—my not wanting oil in my food, dressing on my salad. The four of us shopped at the American markets, filling the hotel room with dietetic jam, rye crisps, tiny wedges of nonfat cheese, talking about our body sizes and where we could get grilled fish. We drove Ilana crazy.

On that same trip I met Mauricio, the owner of the only candy store at the time in Cabo San Lucas. In a drunken stupor I told him my ultimate fantasy, to run wild through a candy shop with an empty Hefty bag. He smiled and dangled a key ring in my face: the keys to his store. That night was probably the highlight of my trip. Did I say trip? I mean life.

What I noticed at Ilana's house in Chicago, though, was how much happier, more connected I felt on my food days. How much more a part of the world. Perhaps that's why I viewed food days as a reprieve, because on these days I could fool people—and myself—into thinking I was normal. On these days I scheduled dates, meetings, social activities. I went out, ate regular dinners (well, as regular as I got: sushi, pasta, salad with real dressing), drank wine and mixed drinks. On food days I didn't think about calories at all, didn't replay the meals I ate in my head. And no matter what, I didn't feel guilty. This was a bargain I made with myself long ago, never to feel guilty for how much I consumed.

The trouble arose when I could no longer control the good days, and instead of eating what I wanted every three days, I did it every other day, and then I couldn't stop. I gained weight. I panicked. I could no longer control my self-control.

When I first moved to New York I would walk around the city, staring at the people in cafés, at bars. Chic and hip, laughing, their forks dipped into each others' sauces, soufflés, their hands brushed against each others' hands while passing bread baskets, bowls of potatoes. But it wasn't their laughter, their clothes, the jewels glistening on their fingers that filled me with rage and envy and sadness. No, what I envied most about these people is that they did something that I rarely could: They ate.

» «

I sound like a nut. I know that. And I was. I was out on my own in the world and absolutely unable to parent myself. What's more, nothing anyone could have said to me—not my parents, not friends, not even a shrink—would have changed my behavior. I was the one in control (or not): *I* was the one responsible for my actions. Unfortunately, I'd absorbed everything, all the messages about food and weight I'd received as a kid—not just the nutritional information, but the disapproval and shame, the obsessiveness, the sense that whatever I was doing wasn't good enough or I'd be thin, as if that mattered more than everything else.

As a parent, here is something you must realize: Just as my parents had no control over me, you have no control over your teen.

There. I said it.

Yes, maybe one day Bill Gates will design a tiny little button that parents can press to program their child according to their specifications. But until this happens, there's a pretty good chance that your teenager isn't going to adhere to your wishes the way you want him to. That's his job, after all, to cause you, his parents, the people who spawned him, grief.

If you don't remember what it's like to be an adolescent, let's try to take ourselves out of our overly responsible, fragmented heads and beam ourselves into the body and mind of a fourteen-year-old. Even in the best of circumstances—that is, if said teen is five foot ten and blonde with a predilection for practicing her viola when she's not studying for her SATs or playing varsity tennis with pals— she's going to have days when she feels like crap, when the hormones coursing through her body overwhelm her, when she hates herself and her friends and her teachers and her life and most of all—*especially*—you. Everything you do bugs her. You congratulate her when she gets her period (Gawd!). You won't let her hang with her friends when she wants to, you won't let her stay out past a certain hour, and you certainly won't let her date. You don't buy her the right clothes, and you monitor when she can talk on the phone or IM her buddies. You just don't get her, and if you didn't suck so bad maybe she wouldn't be so insolent.

Now add thirty or sixty or a hundred pounds to her frame. And take her height down a few notches. And remove some of the drive and ambition. This girl is sensitive. Scared. She wants to look like the other kids and shop like them and eat the same things they do. Belonging to a peer group is infinitely more important than pleasing you. She knows she's fat—how could she not?—and she knows how much this upsets you. (Although, now that you think about it, maybe *your* girth upsets *her.* Ever think of that?) She would like nothing more than to lose weight, except, damn it, nothing tastes better than a vanilla milkshake, cheeseburger, and fries with her friends. (Assuming she has friends, and even if she doesn't—especially then—nothing tastes as good as a vanilla milkshake, cheeseburger, and fries.)

Of course, she'll be self-conscious about this, eating in front of her friends. When you're fat, eating with peers—no matter who they are—poses unique challenges. On the one hand, she might feel like everyone's watching what she puts in her mouth. And they just might be. Or maybe she feels they're encouraging her to stuff her face, that they *want* her to stay fat, because they're just as insecure and unhappy as she is and a fat kid only makes them feel better about themselves. If she *doesn't* join in the pizza party, maybe she'll feel like everyone will think there's something wrong with her (that is, she's on a diet, and thus admitting that she's got a weight problem). If she *does* indulge, then everyone will take note and later dissect how much she consumed. ("Did you see how many Munchkins she ate? No wonder she's such a pig!")

Now plug yourself into the mix. She knows just how disapproving you are of her size, even if you yourself have a weight problem. Not only does she not want to eat with her schoolmates, she doesn't want to eat in front of *you,* either. This sets up a rather unpleasant conundrum: To eat, or not to eat. And where? And with whom? It's not surprising that she'd hide food, or make the rounds of Dunkin' Donuts by herself. It's just too painful to eat with other people.

By now you're probably getting the picture: Adolescence can be a miserable time. You have to have a mighty strong constitution to tolerate high school; teenagers, as far as I'm concerned, are too young to deal with all the pettiness and meanness and drama in a high-school setting. (I also believe most of us spend the rest of our lives either compensating for or trying to reproduce our high-school experiences. I know exactly which people from my past I'd like to see miserable, broke, and alone.)

Teenagers deal with all sorts of issues: psychological, emotional, physical, and, of course, hormonal. And they do so precisely at the time when what they're supposed to be doing, developmentally, is establishing an identity separate from the people most eager to guide them through the complexity, their parents. For a teen dealing with a weight problem, each of these factors can be a hurdle between the desire to be thinner and the ability to appropriately and consistently manage their own behavior.

Let's start with hormones. Just think about all of them that have been lying dormant in their systems that suddenly barge in like Storm Troopers: insulin, cortisol, estrogen, progesterone, and testosterone, to name a few. They all contribute to their condescension and irritation and mood swings and conflicting thoughts and instability and identity crises. They're the reason why one minute your kids are your best friend, and the next minute they hate you. Hormones affect appetite, energy, mood, and concentration, and the unpredictable stew of them during adolescence may make a task as challenging and one requiring as much effort and discipline as dieting seem even more impossible.

As Dr. Erika Schwartz writes in her book, *The Teen Weight-Loss Solution* (HarperCollins, 2004), "Teens are at the beginning of life's journey. Their hormone balance isn't synchronized yet, and they are subject to significant and frequent fluctuations that present often as confusing and sometimes disturbing physical and behavioral changes. Teens and their hormones need to adjust to each other. It takes time to get to the adult configuration of hormone balance that works."

There are also biological factors. As puberty sets in parents may discover that their kids have not managed to elude heredity. Body shape, metabolic rate, and a predisposition toward being overweight, and even character traits that might affect behavior—like, say, an interest or disinterest in athletics—all are heavily influenced, if not completely determined, by genetic makeup. Some overweight kids may have inherited a family legacy of insulin resistance or diabetes.

Kids overeat for a variety of reasons, some of which include hormonal imbalances, or because they're insulin resistant and don't experience satiety. Often, fat begets fat, that is, the bigger you are, the heavier you stay. But honestly, even the experts aren't completely sure why kids get fat, and why some people are predisposed to weight gain. As a parent, it's your job to try to figure out what exactly is the culprit, as Lisa Williams has with her daughter.

"I knew Emily overate, but it didn't seem to me she overate enough to be the weight she was," says Williams. "But it wasn't until I e-mailed a hospital Web site asking about childhood obesity programs that I found a doctor who recognized what I was describing and who eventually diagnosed her as insulin resistant. I thought insulin resistance was something you 'caught' from being fat, but he explained that it is an inherited tendency—Emily's grandfather and all of his siblings are diabetic, so I guess that's where it comes from. It means that her body doesn't process carbohydrates normally, so eating too much fat wasn't the problem, it was too much carbohydrate. That made a big difference in how I had to approach things. Low-fat treats could still have a boggling amount of sugar grams, for example. Pasta with plain marinara sauce was a big treat for me and still okay on a Weight Watchers program, but the pasta had 40 grams of carbs that Emily's body didn't know what to do with. I'd been trying to change how our family ate, but I'd changed it in entirely the wrong way."

The doctor also explained how insulin resistance affected her daughter's ability actually to control what she ate. "It's hard for her to feel full. That's a symptom of the physical disorder. He said her body works chemically like a grizzly bear's, eating insatiably and storing enough fat to make it through hibernation, only of course then she doesn't get to hibernate. So it's much more difficult for Emily to regulate eating because there are no internal signals of 'enough is enough' and there's a constant urgency to eat. That's awful for her, but knowing it is consoling, too. It helps explain why this has been so difficult for her and for me. And it sort of pisses me off that we went for years without anyone getting it, and both of us feeling like failures in our own way because she wasn't losing weight. Now it's still hard, but at least we know what we're up against and what Emily needs to do. Whether or not she does it is still up to her, but at least we're in the ballpark about what exactly she needs to do to help herself."

Other biological factors come into play as well. John Blundell, research chair in psychobiology and chair of the department of psychology at the University of Leeds, in England, has studied whether eating fat can influence appetite regulatory mechanisms themselves. He believes that fat delivers such a dense calorie load that it overwhelms the body's system to sense satiety. "Exposure to fat induces a liking for fat, and people can eat a huge amount of the stuff before inhibitory signaling systems come into effect to stop eating," he says. "Some people are able to eat 1,350 calories of fat in one sitting. Eating fat doesn't stimulate the fat-induced satiety signals but they do inhibit eating sufficiently to reduce calorie intake from the calorie dense fatty foods. However, we're not dealing with a biological inevitability here; some people are better able to tolerate a high-fat diet than are others. These people can eat and stay lean."

Some researchers believe that people gain weight because they don't produce enough of the hormone PYY (peptide YY 3-36), which the intestines release after eating and signals fullness. Overweight people are typically PYY deficient, says Dr. Stephen R. Bloom, a professor of endocrinology at Hammersmith Hospital at Imperial College School of Medicine, in London. But if they're given PYY infusions they eat less. What's more, people who've had gastric bypass surgery often have incredibly high PYY levels.

But some bodies, it seems, truly are resistant to exercise—like, apparently, Anamarie Regino's. They can Stairmaster until they're blue in the face, and it will have little impact on their appearance or physical condition.

In one study, Dr. Claude Bouchard, the director of the Pennington Biomedical Research Center in Baton Rouge, Louisiana, placed 742 people from 213 families through a rigorous twenty-week endurance-training program. None of them had exercised regularly during the previous six months. Bouchard gradually increased their exercise so that by the last six weeks they were exercising three times a week for 50 minutes at 75 percent of the maximum output they were capable of before the study began. Some of the subjects were more trainable than others, while others showed no improvement at all in terms of cardiac output, blood pressure, heart rate, and other markers of fitness. The impact of exercise on insulin sensitivity—a sign of risk for diabetes and heart disease—also varied. Fifty-eight percent of the volunteers got better post-exercise, whereas 42 percent showed no improvement. In some instances, their condition worsened. "There is astounding variation in the response to exercise. The vast majority will benefit in some way, but there will be a minority who will not benefit at all," he says.

» «

Then there are psychological and emotional reasons why kids overeat. "Compulsive eating is for the most part eating that's done not in response to physical hunger but in response to a craving," says Dr. Sharon K. Farber, who has been treating children, adolescents, and adults with eating problems for over thirty years. She runs eating-disorder support groups in her practice in Hastings-on-Hudson, New York. "Or it's a way of distracting oneself from some unpleasant feelings that are starting to emerge—sadness, anger, or a sense of loss or anxiety. Often, many people associate an empty stomach with feeling empty and sad inside, and to them the solution is to fill the emptiness very literally with comfort and food.

You can call it emotional eating—eating for emotional reasons un-related to physical hunger.

"Every obese person I've ever known, personally or profession-ally, eats a whole lot more than they think they do, often when they're not even aware that they're eating," she adds. "They're around food and they grab it and it doesn't even register in their brain that, 'Hey, I just ate three cookies.'"

Farber's goal is to teach people to develop a different relation-ship with food, so they can tolerate their emotions and don't have to self-medicate with food. "Eating can serve a self-soothing func-tion to regulate anxiety, and also a defense," she says.

She recommends that parents not label *any* foods bad. "In the program I run, no food is forbidden—nothing. The women will say, 'If I allow myself to eat Twinkies, I'll eat a whole box and can't stop at one.' They start to dream of Twinkies, hallucinate Twinkies. It's a very simple principle—forbidden food tastes better. That's true with food and with sex. If it's ruled out, you tend to want it more.

"I say to them, 'Buy one Twinkie, put it on a plate, eat it like a regular person, not in the dark, or standing up, or in the bathroom. Eat it in front of somebody or as if you were in front of somebody. Allow yourself to sit down with a knife and fork. If you want milk or coffee or tea or whatever—drink it slowly and let yourself really taste what you're eating.' Most compulsive eaters eat so quickly that they really do not enjoy the food. They may like the first bite, but after that they barely taste what they're eating. I have seen women break out in a cold sweat; they think I am out of my mind. But when they come back they're astounded that they could do it."

» «

Finally, there is the addictive piece. Lots of people I know, of all ages, swear that they're addicted to food, that they just can't con-tain themselves when they're around certain foods: the gooey peanut butter brownie; the juicy Whopper; the butterscotch sun-dae or crisp slice of bacon. I understand it; I cannot for the life of me get off Diet Coke. And when I've got sugar on the brain . . . you'd best not get in my way.

Most experts I've spoken to believe there is such a thing as a psychological, but not a physiological, addiction. That is, they believe we're addicted to the act of putting food in our mouth—we might salivate at the opening pop of a Diet Coke (very Pavlovian) and we might crave a Devil Dog, but we don't actually *need* them.

Something about that never quite sat right with me, at least from my own experience. The underlying beliefs of Food Addicts Anonymous is that sugar and starch-based foods, wheat and flour, refined carbohydrates, are addictive. They recommend abstaining from sugar, sweets, and all forms of flour. As Kay Sheppard notes in her book *Food Addiction* (Health Communications, 1993 rev.), that includes "all forms of alcohol, cocoa, chocolate, 'sugar free' candy, 'sugar free' pudding, 'sugar free' frozen desserts, nuts, caffeine, fried food, salty snack foods, butter, cream cheese, hard cheese, bananas, all exotic fruits and dried fruits, dates, figs and raisins." Apparently one should subsist on air.

But new evidence seems to support the claim that you can be physiologically addicted to food—and that, contrary to popular opinion, an inability to exert willpower over food has nothing to do with moral failing. In fact, many scientists believe willpower doesn't exist. Instead, it's all about "brain chemicals, behavioral conditioning, hormones, heredity and the powerful influence of habits," Jane Fritsch writes in an October 1999 *New York Times* article.

"There is no magical stuff inside of you called willpower that should somehow override nature," says Dr. James C. Rosen, a professor of psychology at the University of Vermont. "It's a metaphor that most chronically overweight dieters buy into" because it lets them off the hook. They can simply say, "I don't have willpower" and that explains why they aren't losing weight. Indeed, it does seem that one *can* exercise willpower, but for how long? That varies. Often the people best able to exercise willpower are those who don't need very much of it.

There are also indications that behavior can affect the brain's chemical balance, and vice versa. "Drugs like fenfluramine, half of the now-banned fen-phen combination, reduce a dieter's interest in eating, making willpower either irrelevant or seemingly available in pill form," Fritsch writes. And Dr. Albert Stunkard, a professor of psychiatry at the University of Pennsylvania who has been studying weight loss for fifty years, "found that people with 'night-eating syndrome'—that is, those who overeat in the late evening, have trouble sleeping, and get up in the middle of the night to eat—have below-normal blood levels of the hormones melatonin, leptin, and cortisol.

"Willpower's role in weight loss was a major issue among scientists about thirty years ago, when the behavior-modification movement began," Frisch continues. "Until then, the existence, and importance, of willpower had been an article of faith on which most diets were founded."

In 2002, Dr. Gene-Jack Wang and his colleagues at Brookhaven National Laboratory in Upton, New York, studied twelve men and women whose average age was twenty-eight. They fasted for almost a day and then underwent Positron Emission Tomography (PET) scans, which gauge brain metabolism. They were asked to describe their favorite foods and how they like to eat them. Then they were shown some of those foods.

According to the PET scan, their brains lit up when they saw and smelled their favorite foods, similar to the brains of cocaine addicts when they think about their next line. The favorite food items most frequently selected: bacon-egg-cheese sandwich, cinnamon buns, pizza, hamburgers with cheese, fried chicken, lasagna, barbecue ribs, ice cream, brownie, and chocolate cake. In the April 2004 issue of the journal *NeuroImage*, the authors wrote that, "Food presentation significantly increased metabolism in the whole brain by 24 percent and these changes were largest in superior temporal, anterior insula, and orbitofrontal cortices"—areas associated with addiction.

"These results could explain the deleterious effects of constant exposure to food stimuli, such as advertising, candy machines, food channels, and food displays in stores," Dr. Wang said in a statement. "The high sensitivity of this brain region to food stimuli, coupled with the huge number and variety of these stimuli in the environment, likely contributes to the epidemic of obesity in this country."

It's interesting—but not remotely surprising to me—that none of the subjects craved lettuce leaves or cucumber slices. "Chocolate is a drug of abuse in its own category," Dr. Louis Arrone, director of the Comprehensive Weight Control Program at New York–Presbyterian Hospital, told *Newsweek*. "It's almost as if people have chocolate receptors in their brains."

In his book *Breaking the Food Seduction: The Hidden Reasons Behind Food Cravings—and 7 Steps to End Them Naturally* (St. Martin's Press, 2003), Dr. Neal D. Barnard, head of the Physicians Committee for Responsible Medicine, a Washington, DC, nonprofit that promotes a vegetarian diet, contends that chocolate, cheese, meat, and anything that combines sugar and fat are addictive. He recommends a strict vegan diet.

Addictions also tend to run in families, which suggests a possible genetic connection. I'd buy that: My mom once ate an entire key lime pie in one sitting . . . which would be a piece of cake for me. Barnard also believes that taste preferences are genetic, which is why some people like bitter while others prefer sweet. I, for example, have never had a cup of coffee in my life; I tried a sip as a kid, didn't like it, and have absolutely no desire for it. My brother doesn't either. But my mother loves it.

Anne Fletcher's two sons, Wes and Tyler, exemplify this point beautifully. "You could put a dish of ice cream in front of my younger son and he'd stop eating it whenever, but not my son with the weight problem," she says. "When they were little I'd take them grocery shopping: the older one would get the most fattening thing and the younger one would get black licorice. That's just how it was."

Dr. Wang has also found that merely looking at favorite foods can cause the brain to release dopamine, a chemical associated with reward and craving. Fat and sugar also calm the brain and lower stress hormones, which is probably why they're known as comfort foods!

"Comfort, of course, is different from addiction," Anne Underwood writes in *Newsweek*. In classic addiction, the brain grows less sensitive to a pleasurable substance, and the addict requires higher and higher doses to derive the same rewards. As Underwood asks, Can food cause that kind of change? Perhaps. Neuroscientist Ann Kelley of the University of Wisconsin-Madison Medical School offered rats plain water or a high-calorie chocolate drink over a two-week period. The animals guzzled more and more chocolate, but produced fewer brain opiates in response. "You see the same thing in rats on morphine or heroin," she says.

Personality differences—genetics—might also explain what makes one child go the anorexic route, like my sister, and another become fat, like me. "Perfectionism is a strong trait in restrictive eaters, whereas impulsive behavior is in someone who binges or compulsively eats," says Dr. Andrew J. Hill, a psychologist and senior lecturer in Behavioral Sciences at the University of Leeds in England, who did his thesis on hunger and satiety. "If you think about how people respond to emotional distress, in terms of eating, it's quite unpredictable. Some people eat in response to depression or anxiety and get mood release from eating. Others in the same situation lose their appetite. That's a really interesting dichotomy."

Appetite varies from person to person, too, depending on one's place on the genetic roulette wheel. In 2002, Brian Wansink, a University of Illinois nutritionist and marketing professor, had student volunteers sit in front of bowls of tomato soup in his lab. Some had normal bowls, others had bottomless bowls that automatically refilled from a hidden tube in the bottom. Those students ate an average of 40 percent more soup before their brain told them they were full. "Biology has made us efficient at storing fat," Wansink says in *US News and World Report*. "But obesity is not just biology; it's psychology. We're not good at tracking how much we eat. So we use cues—we eat until the plate is empty, or the soup is gone, or the TV show is over."

Barnard swears that it's possible to retrain your taste buds, and that they have "taste thermostats" for fat, sugar, and salt. "If you eat much less fat, as in going from whole to skim milk, your fat thermostat shifts to prefer the foods you've consumed over the past five to six days or thereabouts. If you reduce salt intake, low-salt foods will be intolerably bland for the first week but will become more acceptable in the second week, and will be entirely welcome on your plate in the third week. Your 'taste thermostat' has shifted."

In his book he outlines a three-week program—with recipes—to deprogram your taste buds. Before making a lifetime commitment to giving up these foods, Barnard suggests you abandon meat, poultry and fish, dairy products, eggs, added oil, high-fat items, fried foods, and oily or fatty toppings. "Your tastes actually reset to prefer healthier foods, and you've broken your addiction," he said, though he acknowledges that some people might falter, as they do with any addiction. And, of course, he wasn't talking about kids.

Maria Pelchat, an associate professor at the Monell Chemical Senses Center, a private research facility in Philadelphia, says that people often claim they crave a certain good for nutritious reasons. So she decided to investigate, placing a group of healthy young adults on a liquid diet rich with vitamins, minerals, and calories. Still their cravings were as strong as ever, suggesting that "nutritional deficits are not necessary for cravings."

This means that chocolate isn't sought after because it has magnesium, but for psychological reasons. The body "drives them in the direction of food, usually food with sugar and fat," said Adam Drewnowski, who researches food cravings at the University of Washington's Center for Public Health Nutrition in Seattle. "I often notice that offices with very stressful mental work and deadlines usually have bowls of M&M's around." Hardly surprising. Sugar and fatty foods seem to create endorphins, the brain's opiate receptors and the legal and natural way to catch a buzz.

Arthur Frank, director of George Washington University's Weight Management Program, agrees. "The idea that nature would leave this system to a matter of 'choice' is naïve. Eating is largely driven by signals from fat tissue, from the gastrointestinal tract, the liver," he tells *US News.* "All those organs are sending information to the brain to eat or not to eat. So saying to an obese person who wants to lose weight, 'All you have to do is eat less,' is like saying to a person suffering from asthma, 'All you have to do is breathe better.'"

» «

So what does this all mean? That maybe it's not your child's fault he's fat. Maybe he's not lacking in willpower, but simply has some kind of chemical dependency on sugar and starchy foods. I know what too much sugar does to me: my moods spike, I run around with amazing amounts of energy, and then I crash. Hard. The next day I'm a lethargic, depressed mess. Of course, knowing that information and actually doing something with it are entirely separate entities. I try to stay away from sugar, but I don't always succeed—I can't really imagine a life without ice cream. And that's what might happen with you and your child, too. You can take her to all the endocrinologists on the planet, and you can discover that she is insulin resistant and addicted to sugar and predisposed to major weight gain. But it's up to her to monitor her behavior. Let her.

5

honey, i shrunk my stomach!

given all these obstacles, some kids and their families give up on conventional solutions and opt for something a little more radical. In weight-loss terms, that would be surgery, the last resort, the most extreme measure, and one that has become decidedly more popular in recent years. To some people it seems masochistic, a cruel punishment we are now inflicting on young people. But to those who have had surgery, it's a blessing.

Ask Lawrence Capici what's the best thing that's ever happened to him in his seventeen years on this planet, and he will say this: The day the doctors cut him open and took out part of his stomach and small intestine.

Lawrence is soft-spoken and timid; he seems as if he might cry if you look at him the wrong way. And yet on April 29, 2003, he acted with uncharacteristic courage. He had a Roux-en-Y gastric bypass operation—that is, he allowed the doctors to slice out three-quarters of his stomach to the size of a gumball.

It was Lawrence's idea to go ahead with the surgery, known as "stomach stapling" in the old days. ("Bariatric surgery" is the technical name for weight-loss surgery.) Like many overweight people, one of Lawrence's earliest memories is of being on a diet. Over the years he had tried everything—pills and diets and journaling and therapy and hospital programs—and nothing worked. At his heaviest, he was 322 pounds at only five foot three. He heard about the surgery, researched it and "presented the idea to my parents," he says softly. Initially, they were resistant—"They felt like it was a bad idea and were trying to push me to do it the regular way"—but he could never *do* it the regular way. They eventually found a doctor, Dr. Louis Flancbaum, chief of Bariatric Surgery at St. Luke's-Roosevelt Hospital in New York, who performs surgery on kids.

Flancbaum explained the criteria to be eligible for surgery: You had to be more than one hundred pounds overweight and have a BMI of 40 (rather than the 35 required for adults). This is also the criterion set by the weight-loss surgery guidelines cocreated in 2004 by Dr. Thomas Inge, surgical director at Cincinnati Children's Comprehensive Weight Management Center. Before, there were no binding guidelines for adolescents; any surgeon could perform weight-loss surgery if the hospital allowed it. Inge called surgery a last resort and said that it should only be performed on kids older than thirteen who've exhausted all other options and who reach about 95 percent of their expected adult height.

Doctors also look for signs of physical conditions or "comorbidities," like Type 2 diabetes or obstructive sleep apnea, which obesity might cause. All teenage patients also undergo a spate of evaluations, including hand and wrist x-rays to test skeletal maturity, and meetings with a dietitian, psychologist, obesity specialist, and pediatrician, who determine psychological maturity.

"It's important for kids to understand what it is that they're committing to: that it's a permanent operation, that there are going to be changes in the way they eat, other requirements to fulfill, like taking lifetime medications, that they have to be the prime mover of this, not the parents," says Flancbaum. When I ask him how many surgeries he has performed he corrects me at once. "It's not surgeries, it's 'procedures or operations'!" he says defensively. He is obviously aware of language's impact on perception. If cutting into someone and reassembling their insides doesn't count as surgery, what does? He has done about fifteen hundred operations—about twenty on kids. A third of his patients are white, a third black, and a third Hispanic.

"They wanted to make sure I wasn't a binge eater before they gave me the surgery—they didn't want me to have the surgery and force myself to eat afterwards," says Lawrence. This wasn't a problem. He says he never ate because he had a bad day or got into an argument with someone. His hunger was a nagging child that was always at his heels, gnawing at him, tugging at him.

"It was more like a constant feeling of hunger and not really feeling full," he says. "I feel like I was a food addict. I've done OA [Overeaters Anonymous], but I never liked it. I'm not really sure why I ate. I'm trying to figure out. My parents battle with weight loss, they lose and gain and lose and gain. It's just a constant back and forth yo-yo of losing and gaining, and that's what I saw with most of the diets I tried."

Still, his decision wasn't just about health. He's only seventeen, and death, even when you're obese, is usually an abstraction. But there were certainly aesthetic and psychological concerns. He was miserable and chronically depressed. He went to an all-boys Catholic military school, Xavier, where he foundered terribly.

"I was having such a hard time with the kids, I was emotionally down and taking several different antidepressants that were geared toward weight loss, and none helped," he says. There was really no place to turn, no support groups for obese kids or even weight-loss programs designed for overweight kids, especially males.

He did go to one group, but he didn't like it. "The focus was food diaries; every day you'd log what you ate," he says. "Everywhere I hear you're supposed to keep food diaries. I found that wasn't really helping me at all. I'd keep so many food diaries and I never saw anything coming out of it. I just felt like I was wasting time."

His weight was like a graph: Down fifty, up sixty, down forty, up seventy. "I used to sit in the house every day, I wasn't speaking to anyone, I wouldn't even have the ability to do what I'm doing now—talking to you. I couldn't even leave the house." When he was sixteen, the year before he had the surgery, he left Xavier and was homeschooled. That didn't help with his weight or social skills either.

Lawrence knew that surgery was controversial, that there were no long-term studies, but he didn't care. "Even the headmaster at Xavier said, 'You're too young.' It's automatically what people think, that you can't have it until you're old enough and mature enough," he says. "A lot of young kids can deal with surgery better than people might think. Because of the emotional problems they've matured to a higher level, because of everything they deal with, constantly feeling so alienated and looking for help."

The surgery has "totally changed his life"—a common refrain among the gastric bypass set.

"I wasn't afraid of taking the risk of possibly dying or having complications after," he says. "I thought being dead was better than being fat. My parents would rather have me living than dead, but I felt the total opposite, because I wasn't living."

He did have complications—an infection that caused his wound to open up and leak. A nurse came to his house every day and night for two months to fill the hole and bandage it. It hurt like hell. But it was worth it.

Once a week he goes to therapy, and he has done family therapy and nutritional group. "After all that I've been through I feel like I have a Ph.D. in overeating and nutrition."

» «

After getting surgery, as he was slowly dropping pounds like someone out of Stephen King's *Thinner* (except those characters were lucky: the more they ate the more they lost), Lawrence switched to a public school in Manhattan. It was completely different from Xavier.

"The kids don't tease me," he says. "I still feel like there's judging going on—'He's the overweight kid'—and I wish I could go over to them and say, 'I just had this surgery, I'm not going to look like this forever.' I still find it hard to socialize, because I still have the feeling that they'll hate me." He weighs 180 pounds now—twenty pounds less than his goal (he's still five foot three). He would still like to lose more.

"I get compliments from my family and people in my apartment building and my friends about how good I look," he says. "It's hard for me to hear the compliments because I'm not used to them. I'm used to feeling so inferior; it's new to me."

One thing almost everyone has asked him is if he felt that all of his problems were going to melt away with the pounds. No way.

"Once you have the surgery you still feel the feelings," he says. The other night, for example, he dreamed he ate a piece of cake, gooey and thick with chocolate frosting, and he woke up in a panic. It took him a while to realize that it was just a dream and he hadn't pigged out.

Since the surgery he consumes small meals throughout the day, and has had nothing with added sugar, since that can cause "dumping" syndrome—violent vomiting, diarrhea, light-headedness, and cold sweats that come from eating sugars and high-fat foods. He eats fruits and protein and drinks a lot of water. He runs on the treadmill for about thirty minutes a day and is slowly learning to lift weights—the same things everyone must do to lose weight. Except now he can do it—and he does not feel the urge to eat anymore, which many gastric bypass patients also report.

The experts aren't quite sure why this occurs, but it does seem that surgery somehow manages to enforce a lifestyle change patients were unable to make on their own. Lawrence thinks it's psychological. "After you're successful and you feel better about yourself that urge to eat sort of goes away. Like when you do something well, usually you want to keep progressing."

Now his mom, who has been heavy since she was a child, is considering surgery, though she's not fat enough. (Not that it matters; many people *gain* weight so they qualify.) She is short and squat and round. His brother is obese, but never talks about his weight and doesn't eat in front of people. This breaks Lawrence's heart, but he's sensitive enough not to say anything to him.

"When I was overeating I already knew it. I didn't need my parents saying anything to me," he says. "We're all worried about him—

we tell him, 'When you're ready, start your diet.' My mother never pushed me. She made sure *I* wanted to do it. If I was upset about how I looked or I was bingeing I always could tell my mother. She would say, 'It's fine to make a mistake, you'll eventually get this under control.' Even though I felt so guilty after eating and doing the wrong thing—just having her tell me there was hope gave me hope."

Lawrence isn't sure what the best thing is for parents to do. "Diet experts always say, 'Don't have that stuff in the house,' but I don't know if that's giving the right message to the child, that *we* can't have certain foods in the house but *other* kids can. If my parents had a lock on the fridge it would make me feel horrible."

» «

Gastric bypass, a form of bariatric surgery (from the Greek word *barys,* meaning heavy), was invented in the late 1960s by Dr. Edward E. Mason, a professor at the University of Iowa. Mason is also founder of the American Society of Bariatric Surgery and the International Bariatric Surgery Registry, which maintains a database of over thirty thousand patients who have undergone surgery for weight loss.

A decade ago only a few radical and desperate people had the surgery. But then TV weatherman Al Roker had it, and singer Carnie Wilson—who screened her surgery on the Internet for the world to enjoy—and suddenly its popularity skyrocketed.

According to the American Society of Bariatric Surgery, more than 140,000 adults underwent weight-loss surgery in 2004, up from about 16,200 in 1992. While there are no official statistics as to how many adolescents have had it, estimates range from 150 to 1,000.

A gastric bypass operation typically lasts between one and three hours, during which time doctors divide the stomach and staple the lower section into a pouch. "The gastric tract is then rerouted so digestion occurs in the lower small intestine, reducing the amount of calories and nutrients the body can absorb and making long-term nutritional deprivation a potential problem," Stephanie Booth writes in *Salon*.

One of the procedures most commonly used today on kids is the Roux-en-Y gastric bypass, which reduces the stomach to a small sack, which holds about an ounce of food. The first two feet of the small intestine are bypassed.

Although the procedure causes enormous weight loss, it also significantly affects the normal digestion process. Bypassing the first part of the intestine interferes with normal absorption of critical nutrients and causes complications related to vitamin and mineral deficiencies, like anemia (iron deficiency) and metabolic bone disease (calcium and vitamin D deficiency).

In 1980, Mason developed vertical banded gastroplasty, a simpler procedure that reduces the part of the stomach that can initially receive food, but doesn't alter the rest of the digestive process.

A less invasive—and reversible—procedure, called laparoscopic adjustable gastric banding (or LAP-Band), is in the early stages of being performed on teens. With the laparoscopic method, specially designed surgical instruments are inserted through small incisions in the abdominal wall. Though it was approved by the FDA in June 2001, it is only available to adolescents through doctor requests.

Ninety percent of patients who undergo bariatric surgery lose 60 to 70 percent of their excess body weight within the first year of surgery. Then they reach a plateau, or even gain a few pounds back.

But the questions remain: Is it acceptable to perform this on kids? Do the results outweigh the risks? How young is too young? What will the side effects be ten years down the road? (In April 2004, eighteen-year-old Warren Allen died ten months after undergoing surgery.)

The mortality rates, at least among adults, are rather high— about one in two hundred adult patients die from weight-loss surgery each year in the United States. Complications include hernias, blood clots, and serious infections. In Texas, eighteen patients are suing their surgeon as a result of complications from the surgery; in

September 2002, Detroit councilwoman Brenda Scott died from it. Her family filed suit.

Assuming you survive the operation and make the proper dietary adjustments, there are still health issues. Patients must take vitamins, like calcium carbonate tablets, iron, and vitamin B_{12}, in perpetuity. Meals usually consist of less than one cup of food, ground up or soft, so they can be easily digested.

Peak bone mass develops during adolescence, and the surgery interrupts calcium absorption, which worries Dr. Sue Kimm, a University of Pittsburgh professor in the Department of Family Medicine and Clinical Epidemiology. "We have no answers, just questions, and I am concerned that we are not even asking them," she told the *Pittsburgh Post-Gazette.*

Flancbaum pooh-poohs this. "These people are at high risk, that's why they need to be treated," he says. "People who weigh what these people weigh, they will not live a normal life." (These people?)

"It's not that it's an absolute last resort, *it's the only treatment that works for them,*" he emphasizes, adding that after a certain weight people's metabolism changes and the body clings to the weight for dear life. "There's not a shred of science that anything other than surgery works. When you weigh 350 pounds dieting doesn't work anymore; for those people there is no evidence that diets or drugs work. If there were, those people wouldn't weigh what they weighed.

"For example, a good result in the literature of a dietary therapy or a drug treatment is a loss of 10 percent of your body weight. If you take a kid who's 280 pounds or 320 pounds and you put them on a diet and they lose 35 pounds so now they're 290 pounds—is that okay? It's not. It doesn't do anything for them, for the social stigma they face and for all their medical consequences. Even if it can make their sugar better if they have diabetes, it's not going to help their back. To suggest we don't do this to adolescents in the absence of having a better suggestion for them is disingenuous."

Even Fit Matter's Julie Germann has recommended surgery to patients who absolutely cannot take control of their weight. "There's a limit to how much you can lose with the best behavioral program and after that you need something else," she says. "Bypass surgery is a great option if you're at the right place where you have to still be committed to making a lifestyle change. Even after surgery you need to exercise and keep track of what you're eating, otherwise you completely circumvent it. And if eating is their coping skill and fills them up that way, then surgery is not affecting the underlying problem. But some people's lives are so miserable that it's worth the risk."

Not every kid thinks so. La Rabida hospital patient Domnique Gregory, for example, says she wouldn't do it: "To me, it's a will thing. *I* did this. *I* ate. *I* was lazy. Okay, now you work your body to lose weight," she says firmly.

Benjamin Weill, the eight-year Camp Shane veteran, says this: "I love food too much to eat shakes for the rest of my life and if one day I eat a little bit more than I'm allowed to I would be in pain for far too long. I'd rather do it myself than do something irreversible."

What's more, as Lawrence Capici discovered, while most hospitals do have support groups for adults who have had the surgery, they offer nothing for kids, so there's nowhere for kids to talk about what it's like to not be able to join the gang for pizzas at night (assuming they even have a gang to hang out with). Dr. Flancbaum says he is formalizing one at his hospital; right now, though, if kids wanted to come "they probably will get the same info grownups would." I'm not sure it occurs to him that most teens don't want to hang out with older folks, and that info might not be what they're looking for.

Some suggestions indicate that the success rates are not as high as reports have claimed. University of Washington researchers found that, of 3,328 patients who had bariatric surgery from 1987 to 2001, 1.9 percent had died. The death rate was 4.7 times higher if the surgeon had performed fewer than nineteen procedures. (The American Society for Bariatric Surgery has since begun a program to identify "centers of excellence" for the operations.)

On the other hand, after fifteen years, patients who had the bypass were more likely to be alive than those who didn't (88.2 percent versus 83.7 percent). Only 7.6 percent of patients younger than forty had died, compared to 15.9 percent of those who didn't have the operation.

While insurance usually covers the operation, which runs about $30,000 (sans complications), some insurers, like Blue Cross and Blue Shield of Nebraska and Humana Inc., decided to stop. In January of 2005, Blue Cross Blue Shield of Florida stopped covering the operations. They were billed $83 million for operations in 2004, and expected the sum to hit $200 million by 2009.

"The whole gastric bypass universe is being driven by one thing only: Money," insists Dr. Henry Anhalt, a pediatric endocrinologist and director of the Kids Weight Down Program at Maimonides Medical Center, in Brooklyn, N.Y. "Hospitals, which have traditionally been conservative bastions, are saying it's a cash cow. No one knows what to do with obesity, let's just do it, even though there's only a 50 percent success rate with adults who have been studied for at least ten years."

That said, he once recommended a 400-pound, fourteen-year-old kid with Type 2 diabetes for surgery. "But let's understand: we were dealing with a kid whose average blood sugar was 700," he says. "I tried everything. He had three operations on his hips. He had paralysis of his stomach muscles because of his diabetes. He was going to die. I tried drugs. They didn't work."

Strangely, the patient only lost twelve pounds. "We postulated that there was signaling in the gut that occurred and was altered as a result of a change in his road map. So, by changing how his intestines saw food, we altered the signaling from the gut to his pancreas and improved his insulin sensitivity and reduced his diabetes. But he only lost twelve pounds. Was it a success or not? You tell me."

Bariatric surgeons would most likely call it a success. Dr. Philip Schauer, director of bariatric surgery at the Cleveland Clinic Weight Management Program, has performed surgery on more than twenty teenagers and hundreds of adults. According to Schauer, about 80 percent of patients maintain significant long-term weight loss. And though 15 to 18 percent will gain back weight, they're still lighter than they were before surgery. Only about 3 percent gain back all the weight they've lost postsurgery.

"For severely obese patients, weight loss by diet, lifestyle change, or medication has an extremely high long-term failure rate—at least 95 percent, probably closer to 99 percent," Schauer says. "The Subway guy did it—but what the public does not know is that for every one 'Tim'—or whatever his name is"—actually, it's Jared—"there are 99 people that tried what he did and are still severely obese.

"Dr. Phil was on Larry King recently promoting his best-seller seven-steps book that will no doubt make him millions," he continues. "His message was generally good but he was somewhat disingenuous by not telling the public that most severely obese people who do try his seven steps or similar strategy are back to their same weight within two years of starting," he says. "In this one-hour program, the word 'surgery' was never mentioned by him, Larry King, or any of the twenty or so callers. One of his callers was a 400-pound woman—it's wrong to recommend his seven steps to such a patient. Obesity in a 400-pound person is a life-threatening problem that has a mortality approaching that of some cancers. No one questions surgery for cancer. The public needs to know how deadly severe obesity is and that surgery is the most effective treatment— but of course with some significant risk."

» «

Surgery isn't the only option available for teenagers who can't go the regular route. In December 2003 the FDA approved the use of Xenical, a weight-loss drug, for adolescents ages twelve to sixteen. The drug was tested in conjunction with a low-fat diet in teens who weighed an average of 210 pounds. Of the group tested, 27 percent cut their body mass index by at least 5 percent. It was the first time a drug had been permitted to treat overweight kids; still, most people who took it for a year only lost 5 to 10 percent of their body weight—hardly worth the risk when you think about it.

Xenical blocks the body's ability to digest about one-third of the fat in any meal. (By blocking fat it also blocks absorption of fat-soluble vitamins A, D, E, and K, and beta-carotene, so you have to take daily vitamin supplements.) Alas, there are several side effects, like incontinence, flatulence, bloating, diarrhea—not very pretty things at any age. To avoid the side effects you have to stay away from cheese and butter. It's also most effective when combined with a low-calorie, low-fat diet (which, of course, would do the trick on its own).

Two other prescription drugs are also on the market for kids, Meridia and Phentermine. Meridia, an appetite suppressant generically called sibutramine, is undergoing clinical trials for teens, but the drug is controversial even for adults. Consumer advocacy group Public Citizen, saying Meridia has been associated with forty-nine deaths, has pressured the FDA to have it banned. Abbott Laboratories, which makes the drug, says there is no concrete evidence that Meridia is linked to heart attacks. Abbott has said that the drug, used by more than 12 million people worldwide, is safe, and that they haven't asked the FDA to approve it in people under sixteen.

A study published in the spring in the *Journal of the American Medical Association* reported that teenagers who took Meridia had an 8.5 percent reduction in BMI, while members of a control group only had a 4.0 percent reduction.

Liposuction—a process in which surgeons dissolve fat deposits and vacuum them out—also used to be thought of as a possible obesity cure. But a June 2004 report in *The New England Journal of Medicine* refutes claims that liposuction can lower blood fats and other risks related to diabetes.

"What this study tells you is that losing fat itself by sucking it out does not give metabolic benefits," said Dr. Samuel Klein, the first author of the study and director of the Center for Human Nutrition at the Washington University School of Medicine in St. Louis.

Klein's experiment involved fifteen obese women who'd had about twenty pounds of fat suctioned from the abdomen—nearly 20 percent of their body fat, four times the usual amount removed.

Ten to twelve weeks after the surgeries, Klein measured the women's blood pressure and their blood levels of cholesterol, triglycerides, glucose, insulin, and other substances used to determine the risk of heart disease and diabetes. He found no improvements.

With figures like that, and the low success rates of dieting, bariatric surgeons say gastric bypass is the only answer—especially for kids.

» «

Dr. James C. Rosser is chief of Minimally Invasive Surgery at Beth Israel Medical Center, in Manhattan. Rosser, who prefers to be called Butch, is intimately acquainted with the surgery—not only does he perform it, he himself underwent it on August 20, 2001, at 7:30 A.M. (people who have the surgery seem to remember every detail, like a marriage or, perhaps more appropriately, a divorce). He was forty-six and tipped the scales at 450. A Dr. Philip Schauer performed his surgery. The fat world is very small, indeed.

As a professional dieter, Rosser had tried it all: Weight Watchers, Atkins, Meridia (he says he actually gained weight on it), Duke, Structure House. But it took surgery to rid him of 157 pounds.

Butch Rosser is lovely and welcoming—the anti-Flancbaum. When I meet him in his office, he is warm and friendly, his voice soothing and velvety. When I tell him how nice he is, he laughs. "I thought you had to be an asshole to be a surgeon," he told me. "And I didn't want to be."

(But he has his own agenda, of course—he wants me to help hawk his book. Does anyone *not* have a book or TV show in the works? I tell him I would be happy to put him in touch with the right people, but when I let him know how much my advance was he shakes his head. "We're going to get much more than that," he says. He probably will.)

"I always tell people that the operation is the first step, not the last step, in the procedure, and what the procedure does is it gives you a chance to help yourself," he says. He is tall and imposing, a gentle giant. I want him to sing me lullabies.

"I've lost 157 pounds and in the last two months I lost two more pounds. The operation is designed for you to lose most of your weight the first year and by eighteen months you stop losing and over the next twelve months you gain about 5 percent back. I haven't done that."

People regain the weight because their body "equilibrates" and gets used to the condition. But he's a "testimony" that that doesn't have to be the case.

Rosser calls the postsurgery period the "Triad of Long-term Obesity Recovery," and outlines three things a patient needs post-surgery: A well-planned physical fitness program, a well-planned nutritional program, and "an excellent psychosocial state of mind, because the pain does not go away just because you lose the weight."

"The pain of growing up fat?" I ask.

"The pain of being in a world where you don't fit," he says. "That was a tremendous onslaught that was unleashed from not only your body but your psyche for many, many years and only people who have gone through it really understand. That doesn't go away with the weight. That's something that has to be explored, and you must evolve as an individual."

His patients are his "therapy," his "family." "Everyone I meet it's as if I've known them forever. I'm helping myself while I'm helping them. It's an unbelievable situation."

Unbelievable, yes. And also slightly upsetting. How the hell does a doctor—a surgeon who works on and with fat people, no less—get so big?

Rosser has thought about this long and hard. He says it's easier if he just reads to me from the manuscript, and so he does. At length.

I won't repeat his tale in its entirety—you can buy his book for that—but the gist is this: He came into the world fat and hungry. Weighed ten pounds, nine ounces at birth. To quell his hunger, his mama gave him something called a "sugar tit"—"a nutrition delivery mechanism for newborns that was made from a small piece of torn sheet folded and filled with pure cane sugar."

"Do you think people can be addicted to food?" I ask.

He nods and swigs a Diet Coke. "It *is* an addiction, but it's not necessarily a physical addiction," he says. "You go through physiological withdrawals, but mentally you become addicted because of the good feelings you receive in the midst of pain. It's so much aligned with substance dependency that I call what I'm going through now my recovery. Not withdrawal. I'm in recovery from my condition of morbid obesity, which had a dependency on food."

"So if the mother eats junk food she can transmit a craving for it to her fetus? Is that how it works?"

"We know for a fact that you establish fat cells early. If you are overnourished, especially in the womb, you establish fat cells early and they sit there ready to explode."

Jules Hirsch, professor emeritus at Rockefeller University, in Manhattan, believes that an overabundance of fat cells is one indicator that obesity may result from the intersection of genes and environment during infancy or in utero, leading to different responses to food in adulthood.

Rosser's father, an ex-marine and a tough disciplinarian, was the principal at his son's school. There were legacy issues, and young Butch was embarrassed by his weight. So he went through a litany of food crimes, stealing it, hiding it.

He held ridicule somewhat at bay by what he called his "double barrel solution: academic and athletic." He set out to be outstanding academically and athletically, temporarily decreasing the pain he felt at being so big. He played baseball, basketball, football. At fourteen he was six foot four, 285 pounds. Not fat; muscular.

And women liked him. He chuckles. "I've been blessed. I never really 'ran around,' but if you're around me a lot I think—even at my heaviest—I offered a woman a substance of advantages that they couldn't find in another person."

He graduated from high school a few months after his sixteenth birthday, and landed a football scholarship to the University of Florida. Then he realized he didn't want to be a football player but a doctor. So he gave up his scholarship and concentrated on studies and eventually went to medical school. At that time he still played basketball, and while he was certainly large, he wasn't obese.

The anxiety and stress of medical school caused him to gain weight. "You get more stressed as you go up from medical school to surgical residency. They gave us free food as residents and so 24/7 you had food and I was a little bit of a chef. I would go down in the middle of the night and they would turn me loose in the kitchen and I would whip up stuff in between emergencies."

"How did the other people treat you? The doctors, the residents? Were you discriminated against for being big?" I ask.

"Everybody wants to stereotype you and say no to you," he says. "I had to fight to prove the stereotypes were wrong. From the time I played little league baseball, they said, 'You can only be a catcher.' Well, why? I want to be a shortstop. I couldn't run until they saw me run. 'You can't play basketball.' Why not? 'You can't because you're big.' Well, watch me. I had to fight to show them that I could play basketball. All my life I've had to disprove the stereotypes, that big guys are sloppy, they don't pay attention to detail, they don't have good hygiene. I compensated but over the years my compensatory capability ran out of gas.

"No matter what I did, no matter what papers I wrote, no matter how brilliant I was, I always had to earn their respect. They always talked about me behind my back until they got to know me and saw me perform. Why should I have to fight for that? Why should I have to fight for that basic chance?

"I have been absolutely on a mission to prove everybody wrong. Just like people like Michael Jordan and a lot of other people who overachieve. You never feel like you've arrived. But if people just gave me the opportunity to earn their respect I'd be all right. Patients would see me and say, 'Oh, he's a big guy' until I opened my mouth and I touched them. Of course, I have lost patients because they've looked at me and thought I was not worthy. The patients that let me touch them and speak to them, the size actually was an asset because they felt safe with this big gentle giant of a guy."

Rosser believes that obesity is a disease. Not diabetes. Not overeating. Not addiction. But obesity itself. "We have the primary disease state which is the obesity, then you have the secondary disease state, some people call them. But still the bottom line runs contrary to what is publicly thought. That this is somehow a satiation of a psychosocial arrangement that is mostly of a person's own doing. Most people believe this was self-inflicted. They don't understand that these are things that are frequently set into play when you're a youngster."

Stephen Ball, an exercise physiologist at the University of Missouri, disagrees that obesity is a disease. "If we call obesity a disease, then anything that reduces one's fatness or lowers BMI would be a successful treatment, such as liposuction or a very low calorie diet, where we know these are not healthy. By the same token, if you don't lose weight with an exercise program but your blood glucose becomes normal, cholesterol improves, then that could be considered a failure, because it didn't reduce weight. Fitness is a more important indicator of health outcomes than fatness."

Ghrelin is a hormone produced by the stomach that's thought to stimulate hunger. Rosser says ghrelin levels in gastric bypass patients are 70 percent lower than in obese patients and dieting obese patients.

"This is part of that disease stage," he says. "You are having this weight problem because you are predisposed to having high ghrelin levels circulating. That is why people can lose the weight with a heroic effort but they can't keep it off. It's an academically proven fact. The only way you can beat it right now is with surgery."

"What about the stories that we read about in magazines?" I ask. "The success stories, the people who have lost a hundred pounds without surgery."

"Follow them in about five years and they gain it back and more."

"But people gain back weight after surgery, too."

"Not like they used to. Remember the pattern. You could lose 130 pounds but then over the next year you're not only going to gain that 130 back but you're going to go over twenty pounds. With surgery you may lose 120 pounds. You may gain back five to twenty and you stay right there for the rest of your life. That's the difference. It's not just that the stomach is so small that you can only eat so much and you stop. The biggest thing is something that I never really experienced in the past and most people who are nutritionally challenged have not: You actually become satiated. That's the miracle of it. Allowing you to become satiated you now have the opportunity to relate to yourself."

It took him a while before he was ready to lose weight, until "the nuisance of having a few extra pounds becomes the dawn of a new disease. That's what people don't understand. Obesity is a disease. When you get to be one hundred pounds overweight it's not a matter of going to the gym or pushing back from dessert—it's a disease. You would not expect somebody to regulate his or her thyroid problem by eating, because you can't. It is a disease. You would not expect them to regulate their cancer by eating or modifying their lifestyle. Why? Because it's a disease and it needs definitive care. When you're one hundred pounds overweight there is no dieting, there is no will that can give you a life-long recovery pattern."

Rosser finally had enough when he developed sleep apnea and was no longer able to drive a car, which is a passion of his. "When you have sleep apnea you can't stay awake and you are dangerous. I couldn't drive long distances and I love automobiles and driving. That got taken away." His snoring, also a consequence of sleep apnea, got pretty bad.

One day he went into the shower and noticed that one side of his stomach was darker than the rest. (He calls that section in his book "The Day My Belly Turned Black.") That darkness was a hallmark of diabetes. That's when he knew he had to do something definitive.

The surgery, and his subsequent weight loss, affected everything, especially his relationships. His wife even has a Web site, DanasHymn.com, that talks about the perils of loving a person who is, as Rosser puts it, nutritionally challenged. ("We don't say fat or obese. We have to be more sensitive.") He has five kids—his oldest is twenty-seven, the youngest, twin girls, are seven—and they all experienced a radically different father: one who was slow and lethargic, the other who was energetic and always on the go.

He admits that he's not sure he's ready to hear his kids' feelings about his weight. "I know there are challenges that they went through and feel and thank God they love me no matter what. I'm still Dad and they love me but I'm sure they had challenges."

"When you decided to get the surgery did you feel like you were a traitor to the fat people of the world?" I ask.

He hesitates and sighs. This has struck a nerve. "I'm going to be honest with you. There was a smidgen of 'Oh my God, do we lose the persona?' In a way, I love to walk in a room and have people look. I was worried that I was going to lose that uniqueness."

"What do you think when you see an obese person now?"

"When I lost weight I felt like Eddie Murphy in the skit on *Saturday Night Live* when he was posing as white. All of a sudden there was a new world that opened up to me. On the positive side of the world, I could get on merry-go-rounds. I could go on a roller coaster. I could drive a car. Also, there was another world. I could sit down with people and they wouldn't act like I had the plague. I could walk on a plane and you wouldn't see people scurrying. There are people who will actually come and sit down with me now on a train where before they wouldn't. I'm now exposed to comments that I know were made about me because I now pass as a regular-size person."

Once he heard a woman say, "Look at that fat bitch." She was talking about a heavy person on the street, within his earshot.

Did he confront her?

"No, I'm past that. Part of that is because I want to hear and feel the full brunt and let them go on and on. When I see a person that is nutritionally challenged I almost have a Vietnam flashback—'That was me.' That's the initial reaction. Then I develop a level of concern and I entertain a series of questions that start with, What if? What if this person doesn't have the mechanism that I have? What if this person doesn't realize the poor mobility that can happen? What if this person doesn't have access to the care I have? I have a little guilty feeling that I have been blessed and I am concerned that this person will not be blessed like I was."

"Survivor guilt?"

He nods. "You may term it survivor's guilt."

"What about when you see nutritionally challenged kids?"

"I see baby Butch. It's a grief reaction because you have lost a loved one. It's really grieving. You're mourning a loss of a friend and then you realize that you don't need the friend and you have to be careful."

Wendie Pecharsky, who had the surgery at forty-eight, puts it this way: "I do believe it is sort of a grieving process. It's like mourning the loss of a friend—food—which was always there before for comfort. It's a lonely feeling to lose a friend. But you have to fill the void with something else—work, love, activity. I do not miss the fat—au contraire—or the way I looked before. I hated that person. Now I feel more worthwhile . . . I feel like I have joined the human race, as opposed to being an outcast—and I am less than halfway to my goal! Just the feeling of watching the numbers on the scale descend; that is a brand-new phenomenon in my life."

Tricia Winfield, the associate director at Camp New Image, knows what she means. "My whole life I was overweight, and then I had the surgery and within the course of less than a year I've lost all this weight," she says. "People treat you differently. You walk into stores and people want to help you and you don't have to worry about, 'Am I going to fit into chairs, am I going to fit into booths.' You can walk into restaurants, you can walk into movies and it's like your whole entire life changes. At the beginning especially—you meet people and afterwards you think would these people have felt the same way when I was heavy? I still carry my before picture around with me wherever I go. My mother says, 'Why can't you just get rid of that picture?' And I'm like, 'I can't.' It's still such a major part of me.

"I always say I'm the same person now that I was when I was overweight. Then you turn around and you say, am I?" she continues. "Am I really the same person? I know I was intimidated and scared to do a lot of things before that I do now without problems. I went snow tubing this winter. I went to the water park with the camp last week and I was on all the water slides and stuff. I would have never done that before. If I'm standing in my room and I look in the mirror, I know it's me, but if I'm walking past store windows or something and I get a glimpse of myself in the mirror a lot of times I look back to see if it's really me."

These are heartwarming and important stories. But Winfield is thirty-three, and Rosser is almost fifty. Should kids have this surgery?

"If you ask me my response for surgery for kids I would say 'selection,'" he says. "I see this neon sign: 'Patient Selection, Patient Selection, Patient Selection!' I'm not sure that the average child is mature enough to handle the rigors and the responsibilities that come with the long-term recovery. What are the selection criteria? We don't know. Then I get tentative because I don't have the data to do the proper selection to make sure that we don't injure a kid. Then my response is, 'Okay, I've got a problem.' I don't have the data but people need help now. What's the middle ground? At eighteen a kid can probably make a decision. All their growth spurts have finished.

"Now, for an under-eighteen, that's tough. Under eighteen I'm thinking comorbidities: blood pressure out of control, diabetes out of control, and it's not some juvenile diabetes. Can't walk because they are so heavy. That person should be a candidate. Not all kids are like that. But if the kid is under eighteen and having life-threatening obesity causes, you do it. To use this aggressively on all kids before the age of eighteen is very, very shortsighted."

"Do you wish you'd had a chance to have surgery when you were a kid?"

He doesn't miss a beat. "Knowing what I know now, the answer is no. I don't think that I was emotionally aware enough to do what I have to do on a daily basis today. On a daily basis I have to deal with not eating like the other folks are eating. How could you deal with that and make the decision? Peer pressure means so much more then and your peers don't have the restrictions."

» «

One of the most startling things about weight-loss surgery is that for so many people it's a family affair.

Joshua Gee, who lives outside Erie, Pennsylvania, was seventeen when he had surgery in May 2003. At the time, he wore a size 4XL shirt and size 48 jeans, and, at five foot eleven, weighed in at 346 pounds. He was insulin-resistant and had back and knee problems. By January 2004, he was down to 200. His mom, Michelle, now thirty-seven, a secretary at his school, had surgery in February 2002, and went from 322 to 202. His grandfather, Ken Pulos, a sixty-year-old retired welder, had surgery in June of that year. He has lost 180 pounds, from 372 to 195. "After I get the excess skin cut off I'll be 170," he says proudly.

Josh was a skinny baby who had upper respiratory infections, and he went days without eating. When he first started gaining weight no one worried because he was so thin. But then it didn't stop.

When he was eight his mother, who had gained fifty pounds during each of her three pregnancies, took him to the doctor about his weight gain. They saw endocrinologists and dietitians. Nothing worked.

When Josh was thirteen, doctors declared him insulin-resistant, and he was told to stay away from sugar and starches. He also took the antidepressant Wellbutrin, but his parents were pretty lax about the food. "I was worried that if I denied him too much then I'd end up with him as a closet eater," his mom recalls. "And I didn't want to single him out if the others were eating something and make him feel he was different. So we tried not to have junk food around the house like most families would. But it was still here. Not an abundance of it, but it was here."

Something clearly was up. His younger brother, Jay, managed to work his way up to 300 pounds (he's six feet four and wears a size 13 shoe.) Interestingly, his mom doesn't think he should go under the knife.

"Josh has kyphosis of the spine, had back pain because he couldn't support the weight; he dislocated his kneecap and that would constantly pop out. And then they had to put him on insulin pills for the diabetes. His blood pressure was running high. So we were dealing with health issues," she says. "Jay is perfectly healthy except for being overweight. I try to encourage him to eat healthier and try not to have the stuff around the house. But it doesn't bother him like it did Josh. He's not affected by his size."

She knows that people question her maternal instincts—how could she let a seventeen-year-old kid do this to himself? But they don't know what it's like to be the mother of an obese child.

Josh was depressed. His schoolmates tormented him. His mom changed his homeroom, but that didn't help. He couldn't sleep, and his grades fell to Cs. He considered suicide.

It's not surprising that he wasn't afraid to take the leap and get surgery. "I was the one who encouraged getting it done," he says.

His grandfather, on the other hand, "hoped and prayed he'd come through the surgery okay."

He did. Not that he didn't have complications. He woke up from surgery feeling like hell, and ever after leaving the hospital he could barely get anything down without throwing up. A week after surgery he went back to Magee for a one-week checkup. It was a terrible road trip. The usual two-and-a-half-hour drive took three hours because Michelle had to stop the van to let Josh run to a restroom and vomit.

A week later, the nausea finally lifted. And ever so slowly, he relearned how to eat. He slowed down and stopped gulping.

By the time he went back to school four weeks later, he weighed 318, down twenty-eight pounds, and could eat a few mouthfuls of macaroni and cheese and lettuce. While his friends inhaled Belgian waffles and sausage, he took tiny bites of peach yogurt. He takes five vitamins a day, which he'll have to do for the rest of his life.

Three months later, Josh weighed 260—down eighty-eight pounds. Now he checks the nutritional information on packages to make sure he consumes less than 20 grams of sugar and 8 grams of fat. He is a model patient—better than his mother or grandfather, who thinks surgery is the greatest thing since Mint Milano cookies.

"I like to eat," his grandfather says. "I'd eat a pizza and then chase it down with a meatball sub. I'd eat after I ate. I bet I could eat ten to fifteen Quarter Pounders with cheese. Now I don't have the taste for it. I used to wake up thinking about food; what am I going to eat today? Now it's not a priority in my life. I don't crave anything. I used to drink a lot of milk but now I don't even like the taste."

Josh has a similar response to the surgery. What's more, people treat him differently both at school and at the Red Lobster, where he is a busboy. Customers who never used to make eye contact with him now smile.

On October 2, 2003, Josh turned eighteen. He weighed 240 — 106 pounds less than he did five months ago, and only sixty pounds above his target weight. He is studying forensic science and criminal justice at Edinboro University of Pennsylvania; he wants to be a detective. He is finally the person he was meant to be.

6

size acceptance:
fat or fiction?

The other radical solution parents have tried is acceptance. Just plain old acceptance. Love thyself, love thy kid.

Gore Vidal once noted that for every year a person lives in California he or she loses an IQ point. But he probably wasn't including San Francisco.

That, as every good progressive knows, is the place to go if you're at all concerned about synaptic losses and social injustices: gay rights, animal rights, immigrant rights, your right to party, or the right to stay fat. San Francisco, along with the state of Michigan, explicitly outlaws weight discrimination.

San Francisco is headquarters to the National Association to Advance Fat Acceptance (NAAFA), an advocacy group for people of size. Joanne Ikeda, the codirector of the University of California, Berkeley's Center for Weight and Health, has been a NAAFA member since 1990. She acts as one of the organization's spokespeople and is often quoted in the media now that obesity is such a hot topic. She has testified on behalf of both Anamarie Regino and Marlene Corrigan, and firmly believes that it is possible to be fat, fit, and healthy. Diets, she believes, fail 95 percent of the time and promote binge eating and obesity—and are the problem. Not fat.

Studies seem to corroborate this (and this has certainly been the case in my own experience). From 2000 to 2001 Ikeda and her colleagues surveyed 149 obese women, some of whom weighed over 500 pounds. More than eight in ten of those who began dieting before age fourteen said they were never able to maintain permanent weight loss.

Julie Miller Jones, professor of nutrition and food science at the College of St. Catherine in Arden Hills, Minnesota, also thinks that dieting can lead to weight gain. "There is some thought that continuous dieting, particularly with rather severe caloric restriction, forces the metabolism to be more efficient—to lose less energy as heat and capture more for fueling the body. And the net result is that it is harder to lose weight and keep it off," she says.

NAAFA wants this behavior to stop, and for "all children to have a healthy lifestyle and grow up to be happy citizens no matter what their size and shape," Ikeda says. "What bothers me is that there's this assumption that if fat people lose weight they'll have the same risks as people at that weight who were never fat. We have no idea if those groups now have the same health crisis because we've never been able to get a large enough group of people to lose weight long enough to be able to follow them up."

Mostly, the NAAFA folk want fat people—not "the overweight" ("Over whose weight?" snorts size activist Marilynn Wann. "I never use the word 'overweight' because that assumes there's a right weight for everybody")—to be treated with the same dignity as their thin counterparts. They want children—especially girls—to not be filled with the same self-loathing and body hatred as, oh, 99 percent of the women in this country. Most specifically, they believe that it's entirely possible to be fat and happy—the tenet of the Health at Every Size movement, spearheaded by Frances Berg, a nutritionist, editor of the *Healthy Weight Journal* and author of *Underage and Overweight: America's Childhood Obesity Epidemic—What Every Parent Needs to Know* (Hatherleigh Press, 2004).

And fat kids should not be crucified for their heft. It's not necessarily their fault. "We can't hold kids responsible for being overweight if they live in an environment that fosters a sedentary lifestyle and overconsuming junk food," Ikeda says. "The home environment makes a big difference. It all goes back to what you value. So many women and girls are brought up to believe that their value is how they look rather than their achievements and other qualities."

Like so many activists in any arena, all of NAAFA's members have a personal investment in the cause. Most have dieted, starved themselves, battled bulimia, or all three, until finally, in a fit of despair, they threw their hands toward the heavens and bellowed, "No more!" Many, like Dr. Debby Burgard, have created their own offshoot organizations.

Burgard is a clinical psychologist in Los Altos, California, and the founder of Body Positive, an organization for plus-sized women, and the coauthor of *Great Shape: The First Fitness Guide for Large Women* (Iuniverse, Inc., 2000). Body Positive is also part of the Health at Any Size movement (www.healthyweightnetwork.com).

Burgard is not antiexercise but she is vehemently anti–weight loss, especially for kids. She fervently believes it's possible to be happy at a heavy weight—you just have to find the place where your body longs to settle if you would only let it. "One of these ideas is to define 'healthy weight' not from a generic height/weight chart or even arbitrary Body Mass Index cut-offs, but rather as the weight your body is when you are living a reasonable life," she writes on her Web site (www.bodypositive.com).

"A lot of the Shape Down stuff is really decent, but the focus on weight loss is the problem," she tells me. "If you took a fat camp and said, 'We're not here to lose weight but to run around and meet other kids you can be social with, people who will let you be yourself,' it's kinda cool. If you could shift the thinking and paradigm of the adults and make it less toxic as an environment. Don't say, 'Your life doesn't start until you're thin.'"

It took years to arrive at this place. As a kid, Burgard was a fast grower and a self-described know-it-all. She was muscular and stocky and intimidated a lot of the other kids. Though she wasn't fat, she was bigger than the other kids, who figured out that calling her fat would stop her in her tracks. "They called me fat a lot," she says. "I remember asking my dad, 'What should I do?' My parents were very psychologically minded and progressive and he said, 'Why don't you say, "Yeah, I know. Let's move on."' So I did it, I said, 'I know, I know,' and it stopped them in their tracks. But it also felt kind of weird to me, like I was agreeing that there was something wrong with me, which there wasn't. We have this mythology—it's not scientific—that we're going to call people over this weight 'pathological' and people under this point 'normal.' I can't think of any other group like this."

She did her dissertation research on the dichotomy between obese women who intended to lose weight and those women who decided to forget about it and get on with their lives. The latter group was more confident, had higher self-esteem, and generally felt more capable in their lives. "You don't know if those people who felt stronger and less conventional were able to give the finger to society or whether the people who stopped trying to diet gained self-esteem because they weren't engaging in some process of repetitive failure. I think it's both."

Okay. But what about health, and the idea that fat can cause all sorts of unwanted ailments?

"There is something happening that's real," she concedes. "We are getting heavier. Our genes haven't changed in the last fifteen or twenty years, but something about our environment is interacting with our genes and causing things to shift. We really do need to figure out if this is pathological; maybe it is. But even the researchers don't seem to understand their own statistics. It's like number illiteracy. When you read these full studies, it's so much less alarming. It's just not so bad. The doctors are working with the sickest fat people, that's what they see over and over. They see the frustration their patients have. It's been institutionalized by now in medical school and training. You try to tell a physician that there are healthy fat people and they look at you like you're crazy."

That's what happened six years ago, after former *New England Journal of Medicine* editor Jerome Kassirer, MD, wrote an editorial calling the data linking weight and ill health "limited, fragmentary and often ambiguous." He was barraged with indignant phone calls and mail.

Paul Campos, a University of Colorado law professor and the author of *The Obesity Myth* (Gotham, 2004), maintains that the current obesity hysteria is a political and cultural problem, and a way to disenfranchise the unwanteds. Fat, he says, is simply not the evil it is made out to be. "Contrary to almost everything you have heard, weight is not a good predictor of health," he writes, citing several medical studies to back him up. "In fact, a moderately active larger person is likely to be far healthier than someone who is svelte but sedentary. There is no good evidence that significant long-term weight loss is beneficial to health, and a great deal of evidence that short-term weight loss followed by weight regain (the pattern followed by almost all dieters) is medically harmful."

"If you take fat people who have all these health problems that have been labeled weight-related health problems and put them on an exercise program and clean up their diet, their health generally improves yet their body weight hasn't budged much," said Glenn A. Gaesser, a University of Virginia exercise physiologist who wrote *Big Fat Lies: The Truth About Your Weight and Your Health* (Gurze Books, 2002), a book that questions many assumptions about obesity. "It's far easier to get people fit than to get people thin."

What's more, many obesity experts agree that you don't need to get down to a normal size to reduce obesity's harmful effects. Losing ten or fifteen pounds might be enough.

Houston cardiologist Christie Ballantyne observed patients, whose BMIs hovered around 41, as they lost almost 7 percent of their weight within a month. Though their BMIs still pushed 40, most of their comorbidities receded. Their blood pressure went back to normal; triglycerides (the chemical form in which most fat exists in the body) returned to a healthy range; and HDL, which removes excess cholesterol, elevated slightly.

"Our knowledge of weight and weight-related disorders has become so sophisticated that it's no longer believed that everyone who is overweight is the same," says pediatric endocrinologist Dr. Henry

Anhalt of Maimonides. "Some people are morbidly overweight who are not affected from their weight. They compensate quite nicely—normal blood pressure. Do they need to lose weight? We don't really know. Not all obesity is the same; patients need to be studied before it's determined whether they're high, low, or middle risk."

Burgard agrees. "Yes, Americans have pretty much gained a pound a year as adults, and that's a big difference but it's not catastrophic. There are definitely fat people who have health problems, and definitely some who binge and have eating disorders, but there are thin people who do, too. Then you get kids not being able to run far and wide in the ways they could, so physically they're just so much more confined. Then you get the lack of opportunity to be rambunctious. We drug everyone who is hyperactive who can't be quiet 24/7. I think adults are way burnt out and they can't tolerate kids going crazy sometimes.

"We need to give kids time to run around at school. It doesn't have to be PE the way it's taught," she continues animatedly. "I love recess—there ought to be more recess! The whole way we do physical activity in this country it's insane. It's a punishment. PE should be physical education. Let's teach kids how you throw a ball or work as a team or how you know what pain is telling you to stop running and which pain is telling you this is lactic acid building up in your muscles. I think health classes could be enormous opportunities to reconceptualize to our kids what being in a body means.

"I'd like kids to see how to have a relationship with their bodies that's really loving and committed, like they would if they were taking care of their horse or beloved dog or little brother. It's not ethical to ruin a person's relationship with their body, and when you tell someone that this aspect of their body is inherently bad and wrong it's like telling somebody their sexuality is wrong. It might be that they're not taking loving care of themselves and that might be a problem and you might work on that therapeutically, and if the person hasn't been taking care of themselves and they are more physically active and have more friends and lower their stress—it might be that their weight will stabilize at a lower place. Or maybe not.

Wherever their weight stabilizes when they're living that way, that's my definition of a healthy weight.

"Look," she says. "I love it that we're having these conversations, but I hate that we're having them on the backs of fat kids. They're totally aware of what their body means to other people and they don't need to hear it again."

Hallelujah, sister! And she's not the only one to feel this way. Thirty-seven-year-old Marilyn Wann, who is 5'4" and 270 pounds, is one of the most visible activists and speakers on the size-acceptance circuit. Wann is the author of *Fat! So?* (Ten Speed Press, 1999), a fat-empowerment tome, and she regularly lectures to school kids about body satisfaction and size discrimination. Wann swears that she exercises and eats healthfully, and that, more importantly, she doesn't care. This is simply her body's size. She hit the schools after hearing stories about fat kids who were tortured because of their weight, like Brian Head, a sixteen-year-old high school sophomore in Georgia who shot himself because he was tired of being teased; or thirteen-year-old Kelly Yeomans, in England, who overdosed on painkillers after kids threw butter, eggs, and other cake ingredients at her home; or twelve-year-old Samuel Graham, of Fort Lauderdale, Florida, who hung himself from a tree in his parents' backyard.

"It's cruel and criminal that the obesity mafia, the people who spread the hatred of fat, the ones who say there is an epidemic of the 'O' word, that they're targeting children," Wann says indignantly. "If someone had tried to make me lose weight as a child I would be hundreds of pounds fatter than I am now. That's what happened to everyone I know who was at a slightly larger weight and whose parents crucified them. We've had forty years of dieting and we're fatter than ever. Kids need someone to have a discussion with them about body and weight and how to live in a body. My parents were wonderful; my mom was fat, my dad was fat as a kid. They didn't celebrate fatness, but they didn't put me on diets.

"At one point when I was twenty-two I was really bored and working at some stupid job as a journalist—I wasn't as occupied mentally as I had been in college and I went on a rice and fruit diet from Duke for about a week and a half and got really grumpy. Now I'm five foot four and weigh 270. I still exercise and eat my veggies and have exactly the same body type as my mother and her mother. I am proud of that. It's my birthright. I was much unhappier in my life at 160 pounds than at 270. I have a better dating life, social life, better friends, and a better relationship with my family. I don't have a lot of rituals of self-hatred to undo, but I have a lot of internalized messages to undo.

"People say, 'I can't change the world, it's mistreating me so I have to lose the weight in order to get respect, a job, dates, to be healthy.' It's not about health; it really is much easier and effective to change your world than to change your size. Becoming a fat rebel is not a quick fix, but every day I do it becomes more fun and more rewarding. It's way more fun and possible to change my world than it would be to change my weight."

» «

In theory, Ikeda, Burgard, Campos, and Wann are absolutely right, and to them I say, *Bravo!* People *are* more than the sum of their parts. We *should* be able to accept ourselves no matter how much we weigh, and we *shouldn't* be treated any differently than thinner folks.

The problem is that the world doesn't work that way. Fat, in this culture, at this point in time, is not considered beautiful; it's reviled. No matter how hard you try, it's almost impossible to believe that you're worthy if you're fat. It's even harder to impart positive, body-affirming messages to your children. The culture simply doesn't reinforce them. Society is much more forgiving with alcoholics and drug addicts. There's something hip and tragic about the long-suffering alcoholic. It's exotic to be addicted to, say, vodka or pills. Very Marilyn. Very Kerouac. But who wants to be Mama Cass? Who wants to die in a sea of Krispy Kreme boxes? (Elvis notwithstanding—apparently, he was surrounded by fried chicken bones when he met his maker.)

With the exception of the fat activists, not one person I've talked to believes it's possible to love yourself fat. A swell thought, in theory, but rather complicated in practice.

Not that progress hasn't been made on the body-love front. This country has moved inches toward accepting larger role models. Movies like *Real Women Have Curves* and *My Big Fat Greek Wedding,* featuring larger than normal heroines, had widespread audiences. Camryn Manheim, formerly of the television series *The Practice* and the author of *Wake Up! I'm Fat!* (Gurze Books, 1999), got to play the part of a smart woman of size who wasn't about her size. Web sites like AdiosBarbie.com, About-Face.org, and Loveyourbody.org are wildly popular; Curves fitness centers, which welcome larger women, were dubbed the fastest-growing franchise in America by *Entrepreneur* magazine in 2003. (In 2004, it was named the fastest growing franchise in history.) The number of locations has grown to more than 5,500 since 1996. Before January 2003, Curves didn't even advertise. Torrid, a national chain of clothing stores, sells fashionable lingerie, low-cut and vinyl jeans in size 14 and above; Alight.com, which targets women sizes 12 to 32, has had a twofold increase in its sales of tank tops, halter-tops, camisoles, and shorts since 2001. Even models are embracing fuller figures. The 190-pound Emme has become the ambassador of Body Acceptance. Over the past few years she has lectured at college campuses and even testified before a congressional subcommittee about the need to help women overcome their problems with body image. (Unfortunately, her clothing line for full-figured gals went bust in 2003.)

Kirstie Alley turned the tables on the tabloids, announcing her new series *Fat Actress* by proclaiming that she'd had a great time eating her way to 200-plus pounds. (Later, she announced that it was time to lose it by becoming a spokesperson for Jenny Craig—leaving *FA* fans poised for confusion but possibly spawning a new series: Formerly Fat Actress.)

These are all good things. Terrific, wonderful, and encouraging. But it takes a lot of courage and self-esteem to go against the grain. "Thin-is-in" messages still prevail. All of the fat kids I've talked to say fat acceptance is a myth, that you really cannot be happy fat. I know that I never could, and God knows I tried. I'm rebellious and defiant enough to have made a concentrated effort as a teenager, college student, and adult, and I failed mightily. Unfortunately, it seems that fat is the one area where I give in to convention—for myself, anyway (other people can weigh whatever they want). The truth is: I feel better when I'm smaller, physically and psychologically. Exercise plays a huge role—I feel crummy if I don't work out, no matter what I weigh—but I don't think I would accept myself if I were heavy and working out. Is that the culture gnawing at me? My grandmother's lasting legacy? Would I feel differently if heft were celebrated rather than despised? Maybe. Or maybe I just like to be smaller.

I love the size activists, though—I love what they stand for and what they've accomplished and I'd love to join their bandwagon if only I wouldn't feel like such a hypocrite. Because I *don't* want to be fat, I really don't. I like when my muscles bugle and my clavicles protrude. I don't need to be sticklike; I like being ever so slightly round, like my hips and breasts and ass. But I don't want to be fat. It's embarrassing to admit, but there it is.

Benjamin Weill, of Camp Shane and MTV fame, thinks the idea of an organization for fat acceptance is hilarious. "People who can't or haven't been able to lose weight if they've tried, who decided that they are going to make everyone else pay for them not being able to? I agree completely—be whatever size you want," says Ben. "But that doesn't mean I'm going to get a membership card."

Lawrence Capici, who had gastric bypass surgery, goes so far as to say that the fat activists are living in a fantasy world. It's impossible to feel good fat—for him, anyway. "I don't really think there is one overweight person in this world that is happy about being that overweight, regardless of what anyone will tell you. Even if they're feeling good while they're eating, and feeling they should be accepted, I don't think the person who weighs 300 or 400 pounds is very happy about himself. I can't imagine someone being happy not being able to physically move around and not being more healthy."

Neither can Tricia Winfield, Tony Sparber's assistant, who lost 170 pounds after gastric bypass surgery. "I couldn't be happy at the size I was," she says. "I couldn't get around physically and I wasn't doing the things I wanted to do. I always said my goal was to be able to walk into any store and be able to buy something as far as clothes and I can. I would not consider myself happy and I could not have accepted myself at that weight."

"Fat activism doesn't work for most people," says Anne Fletcher, the author and dietitian. "It's impossible to live in this world and be happy with yourself as a person who is significantly overweight." And what about the idea that you can be heavy and a specimen of muscle and well-being at the same time? "Most fat people are not fit and you can't get them to exercise."

Fat activists, of course, don't see it that way. "I'm not trying to change wanting to lose weight," insists Pat Lyons, who coauthored *Great Shape* with Debby Burgard. A nurse in Oakland, California, with a Masters in psychology, Lyons runs the Great Shape camp for plus-sized girls in grades six through nine. It's a place where they can go and exercise without fear of embarrassment. She developed the program based on the principles of sports psychology. "They have a whole world that says, 'Being fat is bad.' I say, 'You can be fat and have a happy life,'" says Lyons. "From the time I was five I was teased about my weight. At fourteen I stopped doing athletics and began dieting and started smoking and by thirty-one I was suicidal because I went over 200 pounds. My intervention with this camp is to give you a model you've never had. My mother tried to get me outside but what was missing was, 'Love your body no matter how fat it is.' That's what's missing: 'Eat your vegetables, be part of the world you live in, and love yourself no matter what you weigh.'"

She cites examples of families who are managing to address these issues with success, and teach their kids that it's okay to be who they are—like Beth Swilling, who lives in Fairfield, California, about thirty miles northeast of Berkeley. Swilling's thirteen-year-old daughter, Shandra, is nearly five foot seven and around 188 pounds, but Swilling doesn't care. She keeps no scales in the house, and she doesn't emphasize thinness as the ideal. It's simply not an issue.

"I don't really watch too much what other mothers are doing; I just know from my own experience and my own history that to focus too much on your weight is a huge waste of time," she says. "I developed really early. I was menstruating by the time I was in the fifth grade, I'm five foot two and about 165 pounds, but I was the tallest kid in class all through grade school. Sure, you can define yourself by what you look like but please balance it out with other things.

"I've always told my kids, 'Look, I don't believe in dieting and I'm not going to help you starve yourself.' I told them the science, that in the end it's just going to get you bigger. But I do say, 'If you think we're not getting out enough then let's do it.' Sometimes we get out and walk the dog every morning. They use the exercise equipment in the garage that I use. It loses its steam after a bit, they're not consistent, but it gets them into their bodies. It's much better for them to listen to what their bodies are saying from a hunger perspective. It's my responsibility to help them to choose the correct things to eat, what's going to be empty calories. But the only time I say, 'No, you can't have it' is usually because it's too expensive."

Instead of bugging Shandra about her weight, Beth tries to probe what's going on internally. "If my kids are self-destructing with anything—drugs, food, exercise—we have to sit down and say, 'What are you not able to express?' There's a cavernous difference between that and what weight you are.

"When Shandra was going through a lot of the 'I'm not pretty, I'm fat,' kind of stuff, we'd have really long talks. I'd ask, 'Why do you feel that way?' and she'd say, 'I'm bigger than my friends, someone's teasing me at school.' My first reaction was to say, 'They see something in you that they hate in themselves, and they're lashing out at you. They have to find somebody else to put it on.' We worked very hard to not take it on just because someone gives it to you."

So far, her efforts seem to have sunk in. Shandra has a pretty good sense of self, and an understanding that the media has caused much of her despair. "I don't think of myself as overweight," says

Shandra, who used to do ballet and now swims and plays the piano and clarinet. (Her mother says she has at least three hours of homework a night, which precludes her from doing as much physical activity as she'd like to.) "Some people say stuff and I shrug it off. I'm like, 'I'm happy with who I am.' One kid said, 'She has mad cow disease' and I just walked away. The media says, 'You can't be overweight' but if they really got to know these people they'd know it wasn't a problem. It doesn't matter what's on the outside. The lesson is: Don't judge a book by its cover. I don't think this is such a big deal. The whole media going crazy about how America has the fattest people and stuff. Yeah, maybe it is true, but who cares?

"I don't weigh myself usually but I just got weighed in PE," she continues. "They weigh us every quarter. I don't see what that has to do with PE; I don't think it's necessary. I just cooperate because my grade will go down if I don't participate. I hope the person who records it doesn't tell everyone my weight! Other people say, 'I don't wanna get weighed, I don't wanna get weighed.' Even the little small people. Mostly girls say this. With guys, the bigger they are the more they like it. Muscle weighs more than fat and some boys like weighing that much."

I am impressed and thrilled by her maturity. She seems to be head and shoulders above other kids her age. And then she says something that makes me realize that despite her bravado and pluck, she's still a kid grappling with the same concerns about being one of the crowd. "I don't want to be made fun of that much. I'm okay with just a little bit but I don't want to be cast out," she admits. "If everyone starts making fun of me I don't know if my friends will stick with me."

» «

If Beth Swilling's approach is political and empowered, Alison Solomon's would probably fall under the rubric of Excessive Mommy Love. Solomon is thirty-two, lives in Dallas and is the mother of four. Her husband runs a computer security software company and does quite well. Solomon volunteers and runs charities, but mostly she's a mom, which thrills her. She is peppy and speaks in exclamation points; I envision her as the quintessential pom-pom girl. She says she's small but has a "big butt."

Her six-year-old daughter, Mary Catherine (MC for short), weighs ninety-nine pounds and is a mere four foot four inches. That's big. Or, in the words of her mom, who is trying to raise a psychologically sound fat kid in an unforgiving universe, "fluffy."

"There's a lot of weight on her," Alison says jovially in a slight southern drawl. "MC's belly is big. People sometimes tell her she's pregnant. I always tell her there's more of her to love! You can't buy jeans to fit kids like her; she's round waisted. So, I buy two and have them redone at the alterations. We tell her, 'God makes us all different for a reason and if we're all the same it wouldn't be good.' MC has fabulously curly blonde hair and a round belly and mommy has a big butt. That's how we approach it."

The rest of the world, of course, is less sensitive. "I love every inch of her but do realize the importance and significance of being healthy. The general populace is not very accepting of overly round children. The current battle is to keep her self-esteem at a positive level. More than anything I don't want people to make fun of her, and they do," she continues. "She started a new school and the coach tells her she's slow and lazy, that she needs to be healthy. This summer we were at the pool where I live—a little private pool for the residence—and my power yoga instructor's son said to my daughter on the diving board, 'Hurry up, fat girl!' She took her time. I told her, 'Downplay it. If you make it an issue it will become one.' That's my motto. Remember to reinforce that you're great, and downplay it with a lot of love.

"My attitude is, 'If you have a cupcake you have a cupcake and then we go ride a bike after school.' MC doesn't have to watch her weight; I have to."

She doesn't know how MC got so big. Alison's mother-in-law is overweight; her husband, as a boy of thirteen, was put on a liquid diet in preparation for his bar mitzvah. He lost forty pounds in three weeks—which appalls Alison. "He was only thirteen!" she exclaims. Her other three children are lean, so maybe there's something genetic going on with MC, who was born "round and precious." But maybe it's environmental. When MC was a year and half old Solomon got pregnant with twins. It was a difficult pregnancy and she was on bed-rest for six months. Ninety percent of the time MC was watched by the Mexican nanny, who took her shopping at grocery stores and fed her excessively. "The Mexicans love their kids; they feed them all the time," Solomon says. "It's very stereotypical of the Mexicans—they're family-oriented and wonderful. They do shower with food. It's a known fact." After that, there was no stopping MC.

(The twins died at birth. Solomon, who is Catholic, looks at it as a positive: "I always wanted five kids; this was how God figured I could handle it. Three down here and two up there.")

One day in October 2003, out of concern for her health, Alison took her daughter to Jessica Setnick, a registered dietitian in private practice in Dallas. This made much more sense to her than shipping her off to fat camp: "If you as a parent need to send a kid off then *you* as a parent need to go! I'm religious; you put it in God's hands and let it go. She might get hit by a car tomorrow and die. Then who's going to care about her weight? Besides, the round kids usually turn out to be the best looking ones!"

Setnick takes a nondiet approach to weight loss. She won't put kids on diets, nor will she weigh them. In her opinion, the key to helping kids lose weight is to "help them find out what made them gain weight and then undo it. Like, if the exact moment a kid gained weight the parents got divorced, obviously he was eating to comfort himself. Weight problems are always a symptom of something else. The idea that if I can solve my weight problems everything will be fine—that's easier to deal with than if my parents are going through a divorce.

"If you eat in a normal way your weight's going to go where it needs to go," she continues. (What's normal, I wonder?) "We don't have to weigh kids—overweight kids know they're overweight. We focus on how they're eating and how they're handling what they're feeling. Other dietitians focus more on what you eat versus *why* you're eating. Like, 'When you're tempted to eat Oreo cookies, go eat carrots.' You can't switch foods like that.

"If someone has a food problem and they don't know which foods are healthy, that's fine," she says. "But there's no amount of food information that will solve emotional eating problems. If you have an emotional eating problem and you throw nutrition information on it, now you have a person who not only has an emotional eating problem but also feels guilty when he eats foods he shouldn't. The solution is to legalize *all* foods, to let kids know that all foods are just providers of nutrients and none of them are good solutions to a nonfood problem. I can help them figure out why they ate that box of Oreos. Sometimes it takes them six months to realize why they got to that point—but the solution is find out what normal twelve-year-olds do when they get mad at mom. It's very nonthreatening to bring your child to a dietitian but 90 percent of the time we'll end up recommending them to a counselor."

MC never went to a counselor, and her mother never returned to Jessica Setnick. MC is still round, still made fun of, and still looking for clothes that fit. Her mother still doesn't care.

7

inner fat camp

an old boyfriend once told me, during yet another one of our never-ending rows about God knows what, that it's the things we don't talk about that are most significant. If we can laugh about something, speak openly about it, then it must be meaningless. But the stuff we keep close to our chests, the things we hide from the world, truly haunt us. Therefore, he concluded, because I made light of my food problems and joked about my weight issues, because I talked freely about fat camp and my grandmother not letting me come to Florida, it must not have been as big a deal as I made it out to be.

He was wrong. People cope with their troubles in countless ways; some suffer stoically, while others derive endless pleasure from blabbing to the world, as Jerry, Montel, and Ricki have so beautifully illustrated. Humor certainly ranks among my favored modes of discourse—and, okay, coping mechanisms—but it doesn't mean that I've actually mastered whatever situation I may be discussing. Though I do talk candidly about food and weight—and yes, even laugh about my craziness ("I can't go to dinner, I have an eating disorder!" "I'm so full—after lunch let's hit the local vomitorium!")—I am by no means free of it. But it has gotten better—partly due to time, partly due to my career, which has given me a sense of identity and self-respect that I was deeply lacking, and partly due to sheer boredom with the subject.

Have I overcome my obsession with achieving a certain physical ideal? Besides wanting to be taller, yes. Sort of. That is, I don't really have food days and nonfood days anymore, and I never, ever step on a scale—even at the doctor's office. This might not be an effective means of regulating my weight (I try on old clothing for that), but it certainly makes me less crazy.

I've also gotten over fat camp. After devoting six summers to losing weight, I simply got tired of focusing so much energy on my body while ignoring what was going on in my head; of putting myself in an environment where I could feel superior instead of learning to feel that way in the real world; of being convinced that my life would be better once I knocked off ten pounds, only to discover that it wasn't.

My last stint at camp was in 1991, when I was at my thinnest and most miserable. That summer my Florida grandmother was dying of a brain tumor and my heart was in the throes of being trampled by a boy named Theo. I was an emotional wreck, depressed and freaked out, and disgusted with myself for being back at camp. While my friends were earning money interning with big-name companies or waiting tables on Martha's Vineyard, I was a Colang counselor, doing leg kicks and arm curls in an effort to reach some unattainable notion of beauty. That summer, one of my campers was a nine-year-old named Rachel. She was tiny and didn't have an ounce of fat on her. One Sunday, when she weighed in only a quarter-pound lighter than the previous week, she returned to the cabin in hysterics. I wanted to shake her and scream, "That's baby fat, Rachel! You're nine years old! Enjoy yourself! Don't end up like me!"

Although I no longer (for the most part) wish that I were anorexic or bulimic, I do worry about my weight more than I'd like to. I don't think you ever get over the fear of blowing up again if you were once big. *The View*'s Meredith Vieira, who is very slim today, has talked quite openly about the 30 extra pounds she carried around in high school, and the havoc that memory still wreaks on her. It rules your life, just like staying clear of booze governs my sober friends' lives. When something goes wrong, my first instinct is to blame it on my weight. It's still easier to tell myself that a potential employer or lover doesn't want me because I'm not a size 2 than because I'm deficient in other ways. And yes, part of me still believes my life will resculpt itself if only I can resculpt my body. Sick, I know. But honest.

I still don't like to eat in front of my family.

» «

One morning in May 1991, my grandmother woke up unable to move her right arm. At first the doctors thought she'd had a stroke, but then they found a tumor in her head the size of a tangerine.

"She's going to New York to see a specialist at Mt. Sinai," my mother told me. "The doctors want to look at the tumor, to see if it's benign. But I can't be there until Tuesday."

"Well, I can," I said, and that was true. I had just been laid off from my very first postcollege job, and I had all the time in the world.

It was spring in New York, and Manhattan never looked more magnificent. The city scared me back then—it was so vast, and everyone was so chic—but that weekend I was not afraid. I was immune to all the violence and danger because I was on a goodwill mission to help my grandmother and tell her everything would be okay, even though somehow I knew it wouldn't be.

I flew from Boston to La Guardia and immediately went to the hospital. It was the first time I'd seen my grandmother in nearly three years. The year before I'd been living with a boyfriend in Key West, and we had driven right past her house in Fort Lauderdale. She'd wanted to see me, but I'd refused. I'd gained twenty pounds during my sojourn down south, I was miserable enough as it was, and I didn't want to deal with her venom.

But she didn't mention anything about my weight this time; she even told me I looked good. That's how I knew something was really wrong.

The tumor *was* malignant—a glioblastoma, about the worst you could get. My parents debated about what to do with her: Should she return to Florida, to a familiar environment, or should she stay with us in Boston? And when the time came, should she be buried with her family in New York, or in Boston near our house?

My mother was firm: Grandma would never forgive her for putting her in a hospital, and frankly, my mother didn't want to. "I can't let her die with strangers, and I can't go to Florida," she said. So Grandma moved in with us. My brother was living on his own, my sister was in California, so it was just my parents, my grandmother, and me.

One afternoon my grandmother, my mother, and I went to see Dr. Cohen, the internist who was looking after her.

"If I do chemo, will I be able to use my arm again?" my grandmother asked him.

"No," he said matter-of-factly.

"Will I be able to walk?"

He shook his head.

"Then give me some pills so I can die," she said.

Dr. Cohen sighed. "I'm a doctor, I'm not in the business of killing people," he said.

I remember my annoyance with him. Whatever happened to self-determination? What about dying with dignity? My grandmother had lived long enough; she was ready to check out. Why wouldn't he do what she asked?

"But we won't prolong your life," he said. "We'll give you something for pain, but we won't do anything to keep you alive. Okay?"

My grandmother, mother, and I drove home, and my grandmother asked me to, "Call that doctor in Michigan, the one who helps people die. Do something!"

Kevorkian was nowhere to be found, alas, so instead I called the Hemlock Society. They sent us some literature that taught you how to whip up a lethal potion, but in the end neither my mother nor I could administer it. In effect, that would be murder, so we decided to let nature run its course.

Thus began the routine of slurred speech and soiled sheets and graying hair and chipped nails and catheters and nurses who cared more about their cigarette breaks than their patients. And, of course, daily weigh-ins.

I couldn't believe that my grandmother was still worried about her weight during the last few months of her life, and I remember thinking: Maybe she's glad she's dying. Maybe she can't wait to be in a place where she'll never have to worry about getting fat and counting calories and fitting into a size 4. Maybe she'll find some peace wherever she's going, away from the temptation of bagels and coffee cake and pizza. Away from herself.

But then I worried. Maybe she doesn't realize it yet. Maybe she's thinking this is temporary, that soon she'll be flying back to Florida to finish the tiles on her kitchen floor, to her scale at Publix, her daily walks, her golf game. Maybe she's afraid that when she finally leaves our house she'll be just another dumpy old lady who has to shop at the one-size-fits-all store. Maybe, I realized, she thinks she'll live. And she'll be fat.

During that period my mother and I often talked about the time my grandmother wouldn't let me visit because I was too fat. We had revisited the subject many times before, but I'd never gotten the answer I was looking for. My mother admitted my grandmother had been wrong and hurtful, but she says she was stuck. "It was her house," she says. "What could I do?"

"What could you *do?*" I asked. And then I stopped because I didn't know what it was I thought she should have done. Maybe I wanted her to force Grandma to apologize (to my grandmother's credit, she did eventually admit that she had been wrong and let me visit for April vacation). Maybe I wanted her to acknowledge that her mother had screwed us both up. Maybe I wanted her to give me back all those years I'd spent worrying if I was pretty or thin enough. Or maybe I simply wanted her to hug me and say, "I'm sorry."

But the truth is, I don't know what my mother should have done. Yes, it would have been nice if she'd stood up to her mother, but it *was* my grandmother's house, and my mother had no say in how she operated. To that end, I don't know what my parents (or, yes, even my grandmother) should have done to help me lose weight. I have hunches, of course, but child-rearing isn't trigonometry; there's no clear-cut path. (Math has always been my most despised subject, anyway.) You can't plan in advance how you're going to handle a problem; you have to figure it out as you go along. One size doesn't fit all when it comes to weight loss. While, say, Hugo might thrive in a highly controlled household, Carl might rebel and become a binge eater. Jessica might be thrilled if you place an elliptical machine in the basement. Erica might resent you for the rest of your life. The point is, *you* know your kid—theoretically, anyway—so to prescribe one method over another seems insincere and unfair. I don't know what your relationship is like, if it's combative and volatile or if it's like the U.S. and England, allies in a war that we shouldn't really be fighting. But I do know this: There is no magic recipe, not low cal, low carb, low fat, low sugar, or low brow. If someone says there's a quick solution, he's lying.

Fat kids are fat for different reasons—emotional, physical, physiological, environmental—and so the road to weight loss has to be tailored to that specific child. What works for Jane's kid down the block may not be the answer for your son or daughter, and the sooner you accept that the better off you'll all be.

Paul Gately has a Ph.D. in Weight Management in Children and runs a weight-loss camp in Leeds, England. "If anyone believes that one skill will effect change, then they're terribly naïve," he says. "Obesity is such a heterogeneous condition—there are so many different people with so many different reasons. The whole process is so dynamic. So, to believe that there's only one model that will work for any one person is wrong."

We all know the technical way to lose weight: eat less, exercise more, and tough it out even when it feels hopeless and bleak. It doesn't matter if you are a pillar of nutritional information. It's all worthless without persistence and willingness, and that's not bred from shame. So, don't shame your child. It's counterproductive. Support your kid, even when he or she falls off the wagon. Respect your kid. Don't demean her for being fat, or for failing to lose weight. *That* perspective, more than anything else, is the problem. The issue here is *not* technical, but emotional. Living healthy is not just a physical endeavor, it's a whole body/mind experience.

Unfortunately, I don't know very many kids who will be persuaded by the health argument. Health is swell, but few of us—of all ages—truly worry about it until there's some kind of issue (and even then, unless it's disfiguring or immediately life-threatening, it's kind of an abstraction). Being attractive is of paramount importance to most teenagers, *not* being healthy. Kids don't care about their cholesterol levels; they care about fitting into a pair of low riders. Talking about the health benefits of weight loss probably isn't going to provide much of an inspirational message.

Change is difficult, and true weight loss takes time. Sadly, your kid is not going to lose one hundred pounds overnight. A dieting, exercising, self-monitoring fat kid is still a fat kid. He might be a smaller fat kid, but he's still fat. But he is working at it, and deserves your praise for that. Focus on the things you love about him rather than just the fat. Your kid, no matter what he weighs, is more than the sum of his parts. And you, gentle parent, need to realize that—and express it to him as often as possible.

(For all of you parents with superior, holier-than-thou neighbors who thumb their noses at you, who smugly proclaim how they would never let *their* precious youngster blow up like yours . . . to hell with 'em. Those who don't struggle with this issue—and there are some, bless them—have no idea of the persistence and deprivation it takes to lose one pound, let alone two or ten or eighty.)

For that matter, not every fat kid is fat because he eats fast food.

"It took me three or four years of the psychologists and the nutritionists and the hospital programs for her to be diagnosed as insulin-resistant," says Lisa Williams about her daughter, Emily. "I didn't know any of that. So all these years I was responding to, 'Boy, are you a horrible parent, you must be letting her eat like a pig,' when in fact there was something physiologically wrong with her."

Kevin Marema, who went to the Academy of the Sierras, ate at McDonald's just as much as his sister, Katie, did as they were growing up. But Kevin is built like his parents, both of whom had weight-loss surgery, and Katie's adopted. Her DNA is different. She's tiny. He's not. She can pig out on Big Macs without any apparent consequences. He can't. It's unfair, but that's the way it is.

How do you avoid shaming your child when an entire society is peering down at you like you're some kind of awful failure for harboring a fat kid? With persistence and diligence and a lot of compassion. It's a process, learning to bite your tongue instead of making a cutting remark. Every time you find yourself about to say something—Bite your nails! Chew gum! Leave the room! Think about it: How many times can you go down the same path garnering the same lame results? How many times can you have the same fight with no resolution? Try to imagine how *you* would feel with someone breathing down your neck all the time.

"You've got to make small steps, and appreciate you can't have this one size fits all," says Dr. Henry Anhalt, the pediatric endocrinologist and director of the Kids Weight Down Program at Maimonides Medical Center, in Brooklyn. "One kid might not lose weight and it might be completely acceptable. Let's take a fifteen-year-old, 300-pound African American teenager who has normal blood pressure, whose cholesterol is normal, who has morbidly obese parents. Should I apply the same rules to him as to someone who's twenty-five pounds overweight? We take each case individually and decide goals for each kid. Changing one's behavior is enough. We don't even stress weight loss; we stress living healthier. It's important to realize that for kids it's pathology, and it's not environment that plays the most important role in why they're overweight," he says. (Although, he adds, 99.9 percent of the patients who come to his office take the elevator instead of walking the three flights of stairs. "If you take the stairs people look at you like you're crazy.")

And what does he think parents should do or say to their fat kid? "I believe that if you don't have something positive to say, keep your mouth shut," he says firmly. "Because you're not going to do a blessed thing otherwise."

Society needs to change. But while we're waiting for that to happen, you can work on the family system. One of the things that impressed me most about Thanksgiving with Kevin Marema and his
family was that everyone knew that Kevin was dieting, but no one
judged him. He sat down at the dinner table clutching his calorie
counter and journal, he ate turkey, vegetables, low-fat stuffing, and
applesauce, and steered clear of the "evil stuff," as his uncle called it,
and he wasn't ashamed or embarrassed or hesitant. That's what a
family should provide—an environment where each member can
work on his own challenges free of judgment and ridicule.

Any change—especially weight loss—has to be emotional as well
as logistical. It has to be a revolution from within. So if you're wondering why Sally knows what she's supposed to eat and why she
doesn't do it, the answer is: Because it hasn't quite hit her yet. She
hasn't heard the click. She doesn't have the emotional backbone.
She's simply not ready—and the best thing you can do for her, while
not enabling her with junk, is to let her be.

"You have to want to be thin more than you want to eat the wrong
foods," says Anne Fletcher, the dietitian and author. "Often in life
we want two conflicting things. We want to be thin and we want to
eat. But the thing you want the most has to give. People in AA talk
about a 'long pink cloud' when they first get sober. After that initial
withdrawal period, that hardship of breaking up with your lover,
there's a period they describe as a sort of superior euphoria. You get
your life back when you quit drinking, you rediscover all the things
you were missing out on. A similar thing happens with weight loss.
When it's new everybody notices, it's so exciting, 'Look at you! You
look like a new person! How thin your face is!' But what happens two
or five years into maintenance? It's deadly boring."

So how do you stay motivated? That's the million-dollar question. One woman Fletcher talked to who had maintained a ninety-
nine pound weight loss for nineteen years told her that, "'When I
was fat, I had almost no mirrors in my house.' Fat people don't like
mirrors," says Fletcher. "Then she said, 'Now that I've lost weight,
every day I get up and look in my mirror and say, "Patsy, you look

great."' What I heard people saying over and over is that they keep a vivid picture in their minds of what life was like when they were heavy and all the things they hated about it. They tell you that they never forget the pain of the past. You could say they're wallowing in the past, but in their next breath they'll contrast that with how great their lives are. They congratulate themselves that they're somehow able to keep that comparing and contrasting fresh."

"Motivation is interesting," says Paul Gately. "For me, motivation is not just about something clicking. There have to be a number of stimuli that allow people to make change. I don't think people just wake up and make change. There's got to be events that make people make change. The kids who are the most successful have basically changed their whole lifestyle. That's far more powerful than some internal mechanism. Also, the family has created an environment where the kids are more active and eat better."

Dr. James O. Prochaska, director of the Cancer Prevention Research Center and professor of Clinical and Health Psychology at the University of Rhode Island, and his colleague, Dr. Carlo DiClemente, codeveloped the Stages of Change model for behavioral change, which arose from their work with smoking-cessation programs. "As we listened to our participants, we became aware that self-changers were articulating distinct stages of change," Prochaska says. "These include: precontemplation, contemplation, preparation, and action, followed by maintenance or termination." Prochaska says that recognizing people's stages is critical to success in getting them to change behaviors, and he acknowledges that behavior change is a lengthy process. One suggestion is to compile a list of the positives and negatives resulting from changing your behavior: *Here are all the things that would be better if I lost weight, but here's the downside.*

"What I've found is that this decisional balance, weighing costs and benefits, continues into maintenance for people who are successful at change," says Fletcher—although she acknowledges that people have to want to change as badly as you want them to.

And even if your child does lose weight, it doesn't mean he or she will necessarily be popular and athletic. It doesn't mean she'll make varsity volleyball or swim her way into a Harvard scholarship or stand at the prom with a rhinestone tiara atop her head. But there's a good chance she'll become a sensitive, humble, and compassionate adult, and God knows the world needs more of those.

Look, this weight-loss business is a lifelong process for everyone involved. It *does* get easier for parents, but slowly. Williams says she has backed off to a certain extent with Emily, but she still finds herself thinking she has failed as a parent for being in this predicament in the first place. "It's hard to get out of the cycle of, 'I'm an awful parent because of this.' I'm experiencing shame," she says.

"Maybe parents'—and our culture's—anxiety about obesity is part of what keeps kids fat, and ultimately, after we've provided all the health information, maybe the best thing we can do for our kids is to truly accept them as they are, and let them go," she says. "Once—and if—the 'click' occurs then it's good to have the information, but maybe the real solution is an inside job. At some level it becomes clearer and clearer to me that I don't have any control over the results and there's nothing I can do if Emily does or doesn't end up taking advantage of the information and help we're getting her. I didn't lose weight until my freshman year of college, as soon as I was out of the house. Maybe when she's out of my house, she'll get that she has to take charge."

» «

I do feel a kinship with the fat activists; they make the most sense to me, at least in the utopian universe in which we don't reside. Their view is the basis of any self-determination argument: *My body, my choice.* Of course, the world doesn't work that way, and it's naïve to think that it would. It requires an enormous amount of courage to swim against the tide. Fat is a moral failing, a cardinal sin in this culture. But the world has plenty of skinny people. What it's lacking is happy, healthy, psychologically sound people.

While some of the size acceptance movement messages are difficult to accept (such as, you can be happy at 360 pounds), some seem more realistic and easier to sustain. Herewith some of my favorites, culled from Debby Burgard's www.bodypositive.com:

- Let go of trying to change weight and focus on supporting solid self-care skills.
- Explore playful physical activity, preferably for the whole family.
- Don't define some foods as "good" and others as "bad."
- Observe the "fat talk" between yourselves and others, and in your own head. What feelings would you be expressing if you couldn't use the words, "fat, ugly, disgusting, bad"?
- Show admiration in front of the kids for people of integrity and accomplishment of all sizes.
- Teach kids how to stand up for friends and form alliances with kids who are being humiliated.

And don't be stupid (this is mine). Don't ship your kid off to fat camp and greet his return home with a freezer full of Ben & Jerry's Phish Food. That's like bringing an open bottle of Jack Daniels to an AA meeting and challenging the members to abstain. Why torture them?

» «

So, what else should parents do? After exhaustive research and endless speculation, I can state firmly: I don't know. But while there's not one easy solution, there are suggestions. And who better to hear from than the horse itself, and its parent?

Danielle Webber, thirteen, offers this. "You're never too young to learn about health and diet, but if I was a parent and my kid was overweight I would tell him, 'I know it's your body. You want to be Miss Florida, Miss Universe, go ahead and I'll help you. If you want to exercise, I'd be happy to help you set up on the machine. You want to eat healthy, I'd be happy to make your lunch. But if you don't want to be healthy and want me to leave you alone, I'll do it.' I would just let them tell me what they want to do."

For her, the way she feels now is the biggest motivator. She says she still wants to lose more weight, because, "I'm loving the way I look now and if I keep losing more weight I'll probably feel even better. When I run in PE I'm one of the top people; I can do curl-ups and sit-ups because I didn't have a lot of weight on me anymore. I have a little candy or ice cream; I don't splurge like I used to. I just say no. If you face something like that you just say 'NO' and it does work. When I'm at school and my friends are eating chicken tenders and French fries I say to myself, 'No, you'll gain weight,' and I think about my bat mitzvah dress. When I'm on a treadmill I think of that and go harder.

"When I'm watching TV and I see those commercials about going to McDonald's to get those big, juicy hamburgers and stuff, I always think I want them so bad. When KFC [Kentucky Fried Chicken] first came out with those boneless honey-barbecue wings, I was craving them so much! But I still haven't had them. My mom and grandpa have a saying, 'Once on your lips, forever on your hips.' I know that if I get a steak sandwich, I'll never be able to burn it off. Once I eat that I'll get so full that I'll just want to sit down and watch TV. So I say to myself, 'You know, it's just not worth it—go get something that's healthy that will also fill you up.' And that's what I do."

Thirteen-year-old Alexis Werth Mason spent a summer at Camp Shane and lost twenty-one pounds in two months. Her life turned around after that. Her mom, Bonnie, is an enormous influence on her. "When my daughter wants to eat, I'm like, 'Lex, burn it off and then have a field day. Eat what you want,'" says Bonnie. "My fear was that when she lost all this weight that she would get so obsessive about it that it would develop into an eating disorder. She's very— 'Do I look fat? Do I look fat?' I have to tell her to stop it. She started eating cucumbers for lunch. From the day she came home I said, 'It's not about leaving all this stuff behind.' The minute you deprive yourself of everything you've loved and enjoyed you will end up compulsively overeating. I've been there, done that. I was trying to create a balance for her and proving to her that you could have your cookies every day but in moderation. If you exercise and burn it off you'll be fine. I signed her right up for Curves and she got on her bicycle and rode to the gym and watches everything she's eating.

"She gets a lot of support from me; when she came home from camp I had these snack bags prepackaged. We're together on it; I cook for her, I force us to eat spinach. I grew up with a mother who was constantly complaining about my weight and yet she had six tubs of ice cream and cake in my house. Lex reads labels and we prepare menus and she's not as obsessive as she was when she came back from camp because I've shown her it's not acceptable to eat cucumbers for lunch. You've got to keep exercising. I say, 'If we're going to eat our ice cream, there's no sneaking. I want it as much as you do and we're going to love it and that's it. Then we'll work it off.' I told her, 'The only thing you can control is your own success. You can control how you look and feel and how you achieve.' She's a straight A student and now she's got her weight down."

Alexis, who goes by Lex, says she started gaining weight in the third grade, after her parents split up. "I was really upset and I just ate because I love food," she explains matter-of-factly. "All you need is a goal. If you really aspire to something, you get it done and you'll like the outcome of it. I want to go to Harvard and Harvard Law and then get married and have my children. I don't want to be a loser. I want to be someone special. I had a bathing suit goal, it was a two-piece and I really wanted to fit into it. After camp, I was scared to eat and I think I lost five pounds more. It was hard: I knew what I had to do, but I saw everyone eating at school and I wanted to also. I know some people who gained some weight back. They just eat, it's peer pressure. But I ate in moderation, and I know what I want and I'm not afraid anymore.

"People don't have time to sit down to home-cooked meals. They're so busy they get Big Macs," she continues. "At camp I learned that there's 590 calories in one. We don't do that anymore. Now, we cook dinners because I'm conscious of what I'm eating. I think I'm always gonna be fat on the inside. We substitute light or fat-free for sour cream; I eat fat-free. There's light everything, fat-free dessert. Even if you do have a cookie every once in a while it's not that big of a deal. You work it off.

"Teenagers have a certain kind of relationship with parents—they have to be your parent and your friend. They need to understand what you're going through. My mother is one of my best friends because she understands everything; she went through it, too."

And for Lex, nothing—*nothing*—tastes as great as thin feels. "Last winter my friend couldn't pull me on the sled because I was too heavy, and I was really upset about it. This year, the next big snowstorm, I'm going to go to his house and he's gonna pull me and that's gonna be one of the happiest days of my life."

Shawn Lowe is a single mom in Los Angeles who's an administration manager for a government agency. She and her son, Zack, fourteen, have also successfully lost weight—courtesy, once again, of Camp Shane.

"Six thousand dollars is a lot of money—I didn't buy anything for three months after!" she says. "I scrimped and saved because I knew it was important. He had no social problems when he was overweight; the only person worried about his weight was him. Back in second grade some older kids made fun of him, and at the regular camp he went to they did, too. Earlier this year I said, 'Do you want to go back?' and he said, 'I don't wanna be in a swimsuit in front of those people.' That broke my heart. I knew how that felt—I was the kid that wore the shirt and shorts over the swimsuit. I come from a family of people who eat twenty pounds of chocolate for breakfast and lose a pound. No one taught me about health or metabolism—I was the only one with a weight problem.

"You can't bug a kid; you don't put children on diets, either. When he was very small I never made him eat just because it was lunchtime or dinnertime. I don't know when I'm hungry. I eat because it's a certain time of day. You see people eating and that's when you eat. I think he knows more about body signals than I ever did. He lost weight for himself. I've always just tried to be an example. I exercise every day, we walk for three miles, it's great together. I never said, 'You're overweight, you have to lose weight.' I took him to the doctor because *he* was worried. At one point I said to him, 'If you could have anything what would you have?' And he said, 'I wish I could lose weight.' I said, 'Okay, let's see how to do that.' And we sent him to camp. I just wanted him to feel good."

"I'm not eating as great as I did at camp, and I'm not exercising as much as I did there—it's impossible," says Zack. "But I go out and mountain board at my dad's house. I skateboard and bike and do push-ups and sit-ups every day. My mom helps me keep it off. She's losing weight too. It's easier when you're with someone who's doing the same thing you are."

How is fifteen-year-old, five-foot-four, 178-pound Rachel Carson doing it? "I'm actually in Weight Watchers and have lost ten pounds already, in two weeks," says Carson, who lives in Amherst, Ohio. "It's the first real attempt I've made at losing weight, though I've wanted to forever. It's working so far, and I sure hope it works out in the end.

"Weight Watchers is a good program, I think, but it's geared to-wards adults. My best friend is doing it with me, and if it wasn't for her I probably would have never done it. I believe support is a key to weight loss. It's so much harder to do it alone. I've turned to the Internet to look for more support, but I can't find a really good fo-rum, let alone an active one, for teens on Weight Watchers. Weight Watchers has the right idea with meetings, but most teens don't re-ally have peers there that can relate. And it doesn't really get down to reasons you're overweight in the first place. Someone has to make a program for teens, and young people; adults aren't the only ones with weight problems. And we have our whole lives in front of us, who would want to waste any more time being fat?

"There are four people in my family, my mom, dad, and my brother. My parents are heavy too, but they're trying to lose weight. My brother's only been kinda big in recent years, and now he's do-ing pretty good because he plays football. I guess I'm lucky that be-ing overweight hasn't caused any real problems with teasing, or nagging, by anyone. Sure, there's the occasional comment brought up by my mother, and sometimes brothers can just be brothers, but

I don't consider it a problem. My friends don't care what I look like, and I've never really been picked on, no name-calling. I guess I'm just lucky that way.

"But there is a person who does care, and nags and puts me down. And that's me. I'm my own biggest critic, and I hate it. I'm the one who always envied what the other girls wore. I've never been able to wear a two-piece swimsuit, midriff shirts, low-rise jeans. I've walked past things I loved in stores, because they would make me look too fat or it didn't come in my size. I just get so angry with myself, like, 'How could you do this to yourself?' And when I look around and see those girls in the lunchroom in their pants with their thongs clearly visible, I think, 'Why me? Why not one of them? Why do I deserve this?'

"I wish I could just have a better self-image, at least a little bit more confidence. And then I would so much happier. I think I'm overweight because I always have been, and never had the impetus to start to turn things around. Until now. I just got so sick of being fat.

"But finally I overcame my self-pity, and decided to reverse what was happening. I just couldn't look at myself anymore without having the driving need to change in my mind. So I did something about it. But I know that weight isn't my only problem, I have to change my thinking too. And that's going to be harder than making the scale go down.

"I would like to know how other kids plan to deal with their problems, and how parents expect to help them. I wanna know how parents feel about their child being overweight—hurt, angry, maybe even ashamed, like their child did something wrong. And I would like to see how parents react to how their child feels about himself/herself. My parents are kinda supportive, my mom says, 'Good job' if I lose a pound or something, but she doesn't watch me closely or dictate about what I eat. It's a self-effort, and I think I'm the one who can really change me. I would like to see my parents being a bit more supportive, but I like being the one in charge of myself."

Amen.

weighing grandma

We do it every day. Slowly she steps on the scale, while the hospice nurse, my mother, or I bend down to read the numbers. It is my grandmother's idea. She is dying, and we do what she asks.

Each day the nurse feeds her three pills—one to stop the seizures, one to get rid of the rash covering her body, another to ease the pain—then sets her on the portable potty. Later, the nurse hoists her up, secures the catheter, and puts her on the scale. There's always a moment of silence until she announces the number, which is usually less than the previous day. This is one of the few things that make my grandmother smile.

One day we get a new nurse, Nancy, who doesn't know how we do things. Nancy puts Grandma in diapers, feeds her Jell-O with a baby spoon, tells her cigarettes aren't good for her health (health? what health?). Nancy doesn't know how to weigh Grandma, doesn't know she's supposed to weigh her at all.

"What do you need to do that for?" she laughs after Grandma asks to be put on the scale. "You're skinny as a rail."

"Because I want to know what I weigh," Grandma says, her words slurred and thick. Her left side is useless, numb, as if someone has injected it with Novocain. "Tell her, Abby."

"It's true," I say, looking up from my crossword. "We do it every day."

Nancy looks at us like we're crazy. "Okay," she shrugs. She untucks Grandma's blankets, raises the hospital bed, moves the catheter out of the way and sets the scale beneath Grandma's feet. Grandma swings her good foot onto the scale while Nancy supports her left side.

"Well?" Grandma gurgles. It comes out *Weggh*.

"Oh, let's see here." Nancy bends down and pretends to read the numbers. "It's about 109," she tells my 80-pound grandmother.

"What? Yesterday I was 105."

I jump off the sofa and head straight for the scale. "No," I say, shaking my head at Nancy. "It's 105 on the nose. The numbers are just blurry, Gram."

"Are you sure?" she asks. "All I do is lie here and eat."

"Positive!"

"You're *sure?* I don't want to be fat when I get out of here."

"It's 105," I say, and suddenly I realize what is happening. The scale is Grandma's link to the world, to power, to life. It isn't fat she fears; it's death.

I spend the whole day with her, caring for her, talking with her. I am in town only for a few days, spending my summer once again at fat camp, my last hurrah before graduate school. I've lost ten pounds so far—the same ten I always lose—and I look good, but I'm not sure if my grandmother notices. I'm not sure what she can see, if she can see, or if the tumors in her head have taken that away, too.

She asks for some moisturizer, and I reach for a bottle. "Do you want a mirror?" I ask.

Grandma snorts. "I've looked at this face for 78 years. I know what it looks like."

I squeeze lotion into her palms and watch as she smoothes it over her chin, cheeks, and forehead. Her face is crinkled, cracked; finally, she looks her age. Her hair—what's left of it—falls in gray tufts around her. Her nails are short and chipped. I understand why she doesn't want that mirror.

Afterwards, she lies back down and I read to her from *Treasure of the Sierra Madre*. She is, unfortunately, remarkably lucid. She remembers the characters and storyline from the previous day. But her attention span is short, and soon she is ravenous. I bring her an egg, bagel, and orange, but she can only eat two mouthfuls. "Aren't you hungry?" I ask, patting her stomach. It stretches tight across her pelvic bones, like canvas stapled to a four-cornered frame. Her bones look like they'll poke through the skin. "Careful," I tease. "You're getting fat."

And she looks up at me and says simply, "I know."

And at that moment it is 1979, and I am back in the seventh grade. My teacher has us fill out forms: *Who is the most influential person in your life? My Grandma,* I write. Hers is the voice of authority, of knowledge. She speaks Spanish, Yiddish, does the crossword in ink. Whenever she comes to visit we bake quiches, play Old Maid, shop at the downtown stores. We only go to fancy places like Bloomingdale's and Lord & Taylor. "Nothing but the best for my granddaughter," Grandma always says, and she means it. Her love is so strong it's vicious.

Today, hers is the voice I hear when I slip into wrinkled or torn clothing (*girls always have to look their best*); hers are the hands that slap my hands when they reach for a piece of cake, an extra cookie (*girls have to be thin and beautiful*). She is the person who wants to know if I have a boyfriend, if I'm writing, if my life is progressing as it should. She's always believed in personal enrichment. She went to college when few girls did, and is the one who wants me to go to graduate school instead of traveling cross-country. "Just get your degree," she said. "By the time you're twenty-five you'll be done." I tell her I'll think about it, but that I might spend a year in San Francisco. By the time I finally do go to school, of course, she will be gone.

I look at her now, paralyzed and weak and helpless. Her breaths sputter, as if a rattler is lodged in her lungs; her bones stick out like pegs. I pat her stomach, rubbing the dead loose flesh, and she murmurs, once again, "I just don't want to get fat."

And at that moment, I forgive her.

appendix

a guide to resources

So many people are doing amazing work around food, weight, and general body craziness, it's almost impossible to list them all. But here are some of the best sources and resources out there, culled by the Society for Nutrition Education (800-235-6690, www.sne.org) and gratefully reprinted and adapted with their permission.

Online Resources

About-Face (www.about-face.org) A media literacy organization focused on the impact mass media has on the physical, mental, and emotional well-being of women and girls. Works to engender positive body-esteem in women and girls of all ages, sizes, races, and backgrounds.

After the Diet (www.afterthediet.com) A Web site designed to help "humans with eating problems."

BBW Magazine (www.bbwmagazine.com) The Power of Plus!

Best Start: A Guide for Program Planners (www.beststart.org/resources/bdy_img/BIreport/httoc.html) Information on planning programs that aim to improve body image.

Beyond Dieting (www.beyonddieting.com) Information on eating normally without dieting and how dieting has affected women's psychological and physical health.

Body Positive (www.bodypositive.com) Created by psychologist Debby Burgard. Includes a host of resources to encourage people to find greater well-being in the body they have—rather than "living above the chin" until they lose weight.

The Body Positive (www.thebodypositive.org) Organization whose mission is to empower people of all ages, especially youth, to celebrate their natural size and shape instead of what society promotes as the ideal body. Includes producing engaging videos and training adult and youth leaders nationwide to help combat body hatred and the early onset of eating disorders.

Bullying (www.bullying.org) Site written by students on the topic of bullying and weight prejudice among youth.

CANFit (www.canfit.org) California Adolescent Nutrition and Fitness Program. Non-profit organization that tries to engage communities and build their capacity to improve the nutrition and physical activity status of California's low-income African American, American Indian, Latino, Asian American, and Pacific Islander youth 10–14 years old.

Center for Weight and Health at U.C. Berkeley (www.cnr.berkeley.edu/cwh) Facilitates interactions among researchers, policymakers, and community-based providers from various disciplines and institutions who are concerned about weight, health, and food security. Promotes collaboration on projects between professionals and members of diverse communities.

The Council on Size and Weight Discrimination (www.cswd.org) Works to change people's attitudes about weight. It acts as a consumer advocate for larger people, especially in the areas of medical treatment, job discrimination, and media images.

Dads and Daughters (www.dadsanddaughters.org) Education and advocacy nonprofit for fathers and daughters. Strengthens father-daughter relationships and battles pervasive cultural messages that value daughters more for how they look than who they are.

Eating Disorder Referral and Information Center (www.edreferral.com) International eating-disorder referral organization based in California.

Fatso (www.fatso.com) For people "who do not apologize for their size."

Femina (www.femina.cybergrrl.com) Online community for women and girls.

Food and Nutrition Information Center (www.nal.usda.gov/fnic/pubs_and_db.html) National clearinghouse that offers information on a range of topics. An up-to-date resource list on eating disorders may be

printed from here. The resource list can be found at: www.nal.usda.gov/
fnic/pubs/bibs/gen/eatingdis.htm.

Girls, Inc. (www.girlsinc.org) Dedicated to helping every girl become
strong, smart, and bold. Educational programs and activities.

Girl Power (www.health.org/gpower) National public education campaign to help, encourage, and motivate nine- to fourteen-year-old girls to
make the most of their lives.

Girl Power! (www.girlpower.gov) National public education campaign
sponsored by the U.S. Department of Health and Human Services. Aims
to encourage and motivate nine- to fourteen-year-old girls to make the
most of their lives by targeting health messages to their unique needs, in-
terests, and challenges.

Girl Zone (www.girlzone.com) Targets teenage girls and addresses a
range of issues, including body changes, self-esteem, peer pressure, physical activity, and diets in an informal and fun way. Girls can learn about the
cons of dieting and eating disorders through journals written in teens'
own voices.

Gurze Books (www.bulimia.com) The most complete online book-
store of books on eating disorders and body image issues.

The Healthy Weight Network (www.healthyweightnetwork.com) Resources and information by recognized scientific experts. Includes authori-
tative, scientific research on dieting, the failure of weight-loss programs,
eating disorders, obesity, overweight, size acceptance, diet quackery, and
moving ahead with the non-diet health at any size paradigm.

Hugs, International (www.hugs.com) Information on the non-diet approach to health and wellness for both health professionals and lay public.

Largesse: The Network for Size Esteem (www.eskimo.com/
~largesse/) An international clearinghouse for information on size-diver-
sity empowerment.

MediaWatch (www.mediawatch.org and www.mediawatch.ca) Works
to improve the portrayal of girls and women in the media.

Mind on the Media (www.mindonthemedia.org) Information on independent thinking and fostering critical analysis of the media message.

NAAFA (www.naafa.org) National Association to Advance Fat Acceptance. A nonprofit human rights organization dedicated to improving the
quality of life for fat people. Has been working since 1969 to eliminate discrimination based on body size and to provide fat people with the tools

for self-empowerment through public education, advocacy, and member support.

National Eating Disorders Association (www.nationaleatingdisorders .org) A wealth of information on treatment and prevention of eating disorders.

New Moon (www.newmoon.org) New Moon publishes two periodicals: *New Moon* magazine (for Girls and Their Dreams) and *New Moon Network* (for Adults Who Care About Girls). The bimonthly companion publications are devoted to nurturing the development of strong, confident girls. Publishes news and fiction for and about girls, without the usual diet, clothes, and articles about boys.

Ontario Physical and Health Education Association (OPHEA) (www.ophea.org) Not-for-profit organization dedicated to supporting school communities through advocacy, quality programs and services, and partnership building.

Partners in Nutrition, LLC (www.partnersinnutrition.com) Listing of services by dietitians using a health-centered approach to nutrition counseling.

Radiance Magazine Online (www.radiancemagazine.com) Online magazine devoted to the positive health and well-being of women. The kids' site extends support to youth around issues of body-size acceptance and self-esteem. Also for parents, teachers, counselors, and health professionals who love and work with kids.

Recovery from Eating Disorders (www.SoberRecovery.com) Recovery-themed resource directory for eating disorders and substance abuse.

Salal Communications, Inc. (www.salal.com) Resources developed by Sandra Friedman, therapist and educator that address girls' and women's issues on size acceptance and eating disorders.

Size Wise (www.sizewise.com) Many more size-friendly resources and information.

Something Fishy (www.something-fishy.org) A comprehensive Web site for information on eating disorders.

Teens Health (www.teenshealth.org) Hundreds of articles for teenagers on keeping a fit and healthy, body, mind, and soul.

Win Wyoming (uwacadweb.uwyo.edu/winwyoming) WIN Wyoming (Wellness in Wyoming) A ninety-member multidisciplinary, multi-agency network in Wyoming and eight other states that seeks to educate people to respect body-size diversity and to enjoy the benefits of active living, pleasurable and healthful eating, and positive self-image.

Books, Pamphlets, and Educational Material

Big Fat Lies. Gaesser, Glenn (2002). (Carlsbad, CA: Gurze Books).

Body Outlaws: Young Women Write About Body Image and Identity. Edut, Ophira. (2000). (Emeryville, CA: Seal Press).

Body Talk: The Straight Facts about Fitness, Nutrition, and Feeling Great about Yourself. Douglas, Ann and Julie (2002). (Toronto, ON: Maple Tree Press). Written by a mother and daughter.

A Book about Girls, Their Bodies, and Themselves. Cordes, Helen. (2000). (Minneapolis, MN: Lerner Publications Company).

Bountiful Women. Bertell, Bonnie. (2000). (Berkeley, CA: Wildcat Canyon Press).

Can't Buy my Love: How Advertising Changes the Way We Think and Feel. Kilbourne, Jean. (1999). (New York: Touchstone).

Child of Mine—Feeding with Love and Good Sense. Satter, Ellyn. (2000). (Palo Alto, CA: Bull Publishing Company).

Children and Teens Afraid to Eat: Helping Youth in Today's Weight-Obsessed WorL.D.. Berg, Frances. (2001). Healthy Weight Network. www.healthyweight.net.

Eating Well, Living Well: When You Can't Diet Anymore. Gaesser, Glenn, and Karen Kratina. (2000). (Parker, CO: Wheat Foods Council). www.wheatfoods.org.

Exacting Beauty: Theory, Assessment, and Treatment of Body Image Disturbance. Thompson, J. Kevin, Leslie J. Heinberg, Madeline Altabe, and Stacey Tantleff-Dunn. (1999). (Washington, DC: American Psychological Association).

Fat! So? Because You Don't Have to Apologize for Your Size. Wann, Marilyn. (1998). (Berkeley, CA: Ten Speed Press).

Fat Chance. Newman, Lesléa. (1994). (New York: Putnam & Grosset Group). A novel for ages twelve and up.

Great Shape: The First Fitness Guide for Large Women. Lyons, Pat, and Debby Burgard. (2000). iUniverse.com.www.iUniverse.com/jahia/jsp/index.

Growing a Girl: Seven Strategies for Raising a Strong, Spirited Daughter. MacKoff, Barbara. (1996). (New York: Dell).

How to Get Your Kid to Eat—But Not Too Much. Satter, Ellyn. (1987). (Palo Alto, CA: Bull Publishing Company).

How to Stay Off the Diet Roller Coaster. Omichinski, Linda. E-mail linda@hugs.com or at www.hugs.com. 800-565-4847 (HUGS).

Interpreting Weight: The Social Management of Fatness and Thinness. Sobal, Jeffery, and Donna Maurer. (1999). (New York: Aldine de Gruyter).

The Invisible Woman: Confronting Weight Prejudice in America. Goodman, W. Charisse. (1995). (Carlsbad, CA: Gurze Designs & Books).

Journeys to Self-Acceptance: Fat Women Speak. Wiley, Carol. (1998). (Darlinghurst, NSW: The Crossing Press).

Living in a Healthy Body. (1995). Krames Communications. Fifteen-page pamphlet written in consumer friendly language promoting lifestyle change rather than weight loss. A good teaching tool for RDs to use with clients. 800-333-3032.

Moving Away From Diets: Healing Eating Problems and Exercise Resistance, 2nd edition. Kratina, Karin, Ph.D., RD, Nancy L. King, MS, RD, CDE, Dayle Hayes, MS, RD, LD, with contributions by Jon Robison, Ph.D., Glenn Gaesser, Ph.D., and others. (2003). (Lake Dallas, TX: Helm Publishing). 877-560-6025 or online at www.helmpublishing.com.

No Body's Perfect. Kirberger, Kimberly. (2003). New York: Scholastic, Inc. Stories by teens about body image, self-acceptance, and the search for identity. By a co-author of *Chicken Soup for the Teenage Soul*. Also **No Body's Perfect Journal.** Thought-provoking questions designed specifically for teens in helping them to think about their bodies in a whole new way.

Nothing to Lose: Sane Living in a Larger Body. Erdman, Cheri. (1995). Also **Live Large!: Ideas, Affirmations & Actions for Sane Living in a Larger Body.** (1996) (New York: HarperCollinsPublishers). Available from Amplestuff: 914-679-3316.

Secrets of Feeding a Healthy Family. Satter, Ellyn. (1999). (Madison, WI: Kelcy Press).

Self-Esteem Comes in All Sizes: How to Be Happy and Healthy at Your Natural Weight. Johnson, Carol A., MA. (1996). (New York: Doubleday).

Setting the Record Straight. Information on fad diets, including low carbohydrate and low fat diets. Includes fad diet book reviews, a side-by-side comparison of the Food Guide Pyramid and several fad diets, poster, and guest column. www.wheatfoods.org.

Size Wise: A Catalog of More Than 1000 Resources for Living with Confidence and Comfort at Any Size. Sullivan, Judy. (1997). (New York: Avon Books).

Studies in Eating Disorders—An International Series: The Prevention of Eating Disorders. Vandereycken, Walter, and Greta Noordenbos. (1998). (London: Athlone Press).

Tipping the Scales of Justice: Fighting Weight-Based Discrimination. Solovay, Sondra, JD. (2000). (Amherst, NY: Prometheus Books).

The Truth About Body and Beauty. Cooke, Kaz. (1998). (New York: W. W. Norton).

Underage and Overweight: America's Childhood Obesity Epidemic—What Every Parent Needs to Know. Berg, Frances, MS. (2004). (Hatherleigh Press). www.healthyweight.net.

Wake Up, I'm Fat! Manheim, Camryn. (1999). (New York: Broadway Books).

Weight Issues: Fatness and Thinness as Social Problems. Sobal, Jeffery, and Donna Maurer. (1999). (New York: Aldine de Gruyter).

When Girls Feel Fat—Helping Girls Through Adolescence. Friedman, Sandra Susan. (2000). (Buffalo, NY: Firefly Books). www.salal.com.

When Women Stop Hating Their Bodies: Freeing Yourself from Food and Weight Obsession. Hirschmann, Jane R., MSW, and Carol H. Munter. (1997). (New York: Fawcett Books).

Women Afraid to Eat: Breaking Free in Today's Weight-Obsessed World. Berg, Frances. (1999). (Hettinger, ND: Healthy Weight Network). Healthy Weight Network: 402 South 14th St., Hettinger, ND 58639. Phone 701-567-2646, Fax 701-567-2606. Order online from www.healthyweight.net.

Worth Your Weight: What You Can Do About a Weight Problem. Bruno, Barbara Altman, Ph.D. (1996). (Rutledge Books).

You Count, Calories Don't. Omichinski, Linda, RD. (1996). (London: Hodder & Stoughton). Email linda@hugs.com. Web site www.hugs.com.

Professional Journals and Newsletters
Promoting Health at Every Size

Health at Every Size (formerly Healthy Weight Journal). Research, news, and commentary across the weight spectrum. Published by BC Decker, Inc. Ordering information available online at www.bcdecker.com. Enter journal title in search window. Membership not required to shop.

Resources for Children and Teens

BodyTalk. Twenty-eight-minute video on body acceptance issues for adolescent girls and boys. Features girls and boys who represent diverse ethnic backgrounds, and socioeconomic status and body size discussing how they accept themselves and reject pressures to be thin. Connie Sobczak, Executive Director, The Body Positive, 2550 9th Street, suite 204B, Berkeley, CA 94710. E-mail: info@thebodypositive.org or visit www.thebodypositive.org for ordering information.

Childhood and Adolescent Obesity in America: What's a Parent to Do? A pamphlet by Betty Holmes, MS, RD. (1998). Twelve-page booklet provides an overview on the failure of dieting, size acceptance, normal and healthy eating, the importance of physical activity, and successful strategies for parents of overweight children. For more information or to place an order, contact the Office of Communications and Technology Resource Center, University of Wyoming: Phone 307-766-2115. Fax 307-766-2800. Can be printed from the Web site uwacadweb.uwyo.edu/cesnutrition/. Go to UW Food and Nutrition Publications, and click on "Healthy Lifestyles/Healthy Weight".

Guidelines for Childhood Obesity Prevention Programs: Promoting Healthy Weight in Children. Developed by the Weight Realities Division of the Society for Nutrition Education, October 2002. Available online at www.healthyweight.net.

Help Your Child with Successful Weight Management. From the USDA/ARS Children's Nutrition Research Center at the Baylor College of Medicine, (2001). Four-page pamphlet provides information on common causes of weight problems in children and offers suggestions for ways that families can work together to increase physical activity and have healthy eating habits. Encourages family goal setting and includes how to find professional assistance. Order free from: Children's Nutrition Research Center, 1100 Bates Street, Houston, TX 77030, e-mail to cnrc@bcm.tmc.edu. Language: English and Spanish. Can also be downloaded and printed from the Web site www.bcm.tmc.edu/cnrc. Scroll down to "Brochures" (below "Search this Site"), then "From the CRNC: Help Your Child with Successful Weight Management".

Helping Your Overweight Child. (1997). From the Weight-Control Information Network, National Institute of Diabetes and Digestive and Kidney Diseases, National Institutes of Health. Information for parents on what causes children to become overweight, how to tell if a child is overweight and how to help an overweight child. Practical suggestions for helping children develop positive attitudes about eating. Provides simple snack ideas. Order free from: Weight-Control Information Network, 877-946-4627 Language: English Cost: free for up to 25 photocopies. Can also be printed from the Web site win.niddk.nih.gov/publications/.

If My Child is Overweight, What Should I Do about It? By Joanne Ikeda, MA, RD, University of California Extension nutrition specialist. Twenty-page booklet for parents on how to help overweight children. Written in a question and answer format, including how to tell if a child is overweight, how to talk to a child about weight, suggestions for healthy food choices, and advice on increasing physical activity. Order from: ANR Communications, University of California, 800-994-8849. Online from anrcatalog.ucdavis.edu/. Click on "Nutrition & Eating Right".

Teens & Diets No Weigh. By Linda Omichinski, RD. Prevention program for schools and groups that confronts the epidemic of teen dieting, body shape preoccupation, and eating disorders. Helps youth develop non-diet lifestyle, adopt healthy eating patterns, live actively, and celebrate their natural body shapes. Eight lessons with complete plans, support material, teen journal, parent guide handbook, cookbook. Recommended for health or nutrition curriculum, community groups. Licensing agreement. Includes "Afraid to Eat" and home study course: Weight Management for Teens. Available online at www.hugs.com. Click on "Take" program, then "Programs", then "Teen Program".

Ten Steps for Parents. From USDA Team Nutrition. (2002). Includes both a Food Guide Pyramid and a physical activity pyramid. Also offers tips for making exercise easy and for encouraging healthy eating at school and at home. Order from: Team Nutrition, order online (see Web address below) or fax your name, address, publication name and number of copies desired to fax 703-605-6852. Publication number USDA9 (English version), USDA75 (Spanish version). Language: English and Spanish. Cost: free to schools and parents. Can also be downloaded and printed either in color or black and white at www.fns.usda.gov/tn. Click on "Resources."

notes

Introduction: Fat Kid Blues

page xxix   **"'Kids live basically in a dictatorship while they are in their parents' home.'"** Michael Fumento quoted in Leibovich, Lori: "Fat People, Get Real!" *Salon*, September 12, 1997, http://archive.salon.com/sept97/news/news970912.html.

page xxix   **"'Your anxiety is that you have ruined the child.'"** In-person interview with Lisa Williams.

page xxx   **"'It was very difficult and embarrassing.'"** Telephone interview with Anne M. Fletcher, MS, RD, LD.

page xxxi   **"The diet industry, after all is a $46.3 billion dollar business . . ."** Statistics come from Market Data Enterprises, Inc., a Tampa-based research and consulting firm that specializes in the diet market.

page xxxi   **"In 2003, Weight Watchers had revenues of $1 billion . . ."** Statistics from Weight Watchers International Corporate Press Office; Jenny Craig Corporate Press Office.

page xxxiii   **"Ironically, about two years ago Weight Watchers stopped allowing children under ten . . ."** Telephone interview with Karen Miller-Kovach, MS, RD, chief scientific officer at Weight Watchers International.

page xxxvi   **"According to the latest federal figures, the percentage of youngsters ages six to eleven who are overweight . . ."** Statistics from the Centers for Disease Control, 2004. Telephone interviews.

page xxxvi   **"A study by the University of Michigan and the University of Medicine and Dentistry of New Jersey surveyed 17,500 adolescents . . ."** Hedley, Alison, and Cynthia Ogden,

233

et al., "National Health and Nutrition Examination Survey, Clinical Measurements in Mobile Examination Facilities, Centers for Disease Control and Prevention." *Journal of American Medical Association,* 291, 285.

page xxxvi   **"A study by the University of Minnesota researchers interviewed 4,746 kids in grades seven to twelve . . ."** E-mail interview with Marla Eisenberg, Sc.D., M.P.H., a research associate in the University of Minnesota School of Public Health and Medical School.

page xxxvi   **"Overweight adolescents are also more apt than normal-weight children to be victims . . ."** *Pediatrics,* May, 2004.

page xxxviii   **"By age nine children have developed an active dislike of fat bodies . . ."** Study conducted by M. Feldman, E. Feldman, and J.T. Goodman, "Culture versus Biology: Children's Attitudes Towards Thinness and Fatness," in Pediatrics 81 (1988): 190–94.

Chapter 1: Ho Hos in Paradise

page 13   **"'I had a miserable Childhood . . .'"** In-person interview with Tony Sparber at Camp Pocono Trails. All statistics and figures, as well as his background history, arise from this interview.

page 22   **"Tony Sparber's assistant director, Trish Winfield . . ."** In-person interview with Tricia Winfield at Camp Pocono Trails.

page 23   **"'I think if I hadn't gone to Shane I'd be significantly heavier than I am and have ever been.'"** In-person interview with Benjamin Weill.

page 26   **"Not quite true, says his mom."** In-person interview with Terry Weill.

page 27   **"Weight loss camps peaked in 1988, with eighty-four camps."** Telephone interview with Lucy J. Norvell, director of Public Information for the American Camping Association of New England.

page 28   **"Ettenberg, fifty-seven, welcomes media."** In-person interview with David Ettenberg at Camp Shane.

page 35   **"'This is my first time in the U.S. and I can understand why** kids . . .'" In-person interview and e-mail correspondence with Sarah Carter.

page 37   "'They don't give a report back . . .'" Telephone interview with Fran Moscowitz.

page 38   "'It's a sad statement, but I feel the majority of parents would rather. . .'" Telephone interview with Lydia Burton (not her real name).

page 40   "Mary Stevens is one of the lucky ones." In-person interview with Mary Stevens at Camp La Jolla.

page 41   "At first, the beauty of Camp Shane overwhelmed her." In-person interview, telephone conversations, and e-mail correspondence with Lucy Walker (not her real name).

page 44   "He has seen two different dietitians, worked out with a personal trainer . . ." In-person and email interviews with Kevin Marema and his parents at Academy of the Sierras and in Ft. Lauderdale, Florida.

page 46   "Craig, thirty-four, spent three years as a vice president at Warburg-Pincus . . ." In-person, telephone, and e-mail interviews with Ryan Craig at AOS and at Camp Wellspring.

page 47   "Actually, there is a program in Germany . . ." Telephone interview with Wolfang Sigfried, clinical director of Insula Rehabilitation Centre.

page 49   "Kirschenbaum, fifty-one, believes self-control can be taught . . ." In-person and telephone interviews with Dr. Daniel S. Kirschenbaum, professor of psychiatry and Behavioral Sciences at Northwestern University Medical School, in Chicago.

page 51   "'These kids aren't as hostile and angry . . .'" In-person interview with Dan Barry at AOS.

page 53   "'They're victims of a culture assaulting them with mixed messages." In-person and telephone interviews with Molly Carmel, MSW.

page 55   "'The mental illness is nothing compared to the extra pounds.'" In-person interview with Stacey Fay.

page 59   "'self-monitoring shows that people are watching their food intake . . .'" Telephone interview with Dr. Thomas Wadden, Ph.D., director of the weight and eating disorders program at the University of Pennsylvania School of Medicine.

Chapter 2: Behavior Modification and Its Discontents

page 61 **"The free program targets lower income and minority . . ."** In-person, telephone interviews, and e-mail correspondence with Dr. Julie Germann, Ph.D., program coordinator for the Fit Matters program at La Rabida Children's Hospital, which is where all the figures come from.

page 62 **"The National Institutes of Health report that 80 percent of African-American women . . ."** Statistics from NIH.

page 67 **". . . who I later learn weighed 220 pounds as a kid."** In-person, telephone interviews with Tina Musselman, RD.

page 67 **"Fast food is very common in both public and private hospitals across the country . . ."** Marc Santora, "Burgers for the Health Professional," *New York Times,* October 26, 2004.

page 68 **"Patients who eat three to four servings of dairy . . ."** E-mail interview with Dr. Michael B. Zemel, Ph.D., Professor of Nutrition & Medicine and Director of the Nutrition Institute at the University of Tennessee, Knoxville.

page 70 **"Around 16 percent of whites who earn $50,000 are obese . . ."** David Barboza, "Rampant Obesity, a Debilitating Reality for the Urban Poor," *New York Times*, December 26, 2000.

page 70 **"A 1999 A.C. Nielsen Home Scan survey monitoring consumer patterns . . ."** Barboza, "Rampant Obesity."

page 71 **"A 2001 study. . . found that blacks watch an average of seventy-five hours of TV a week . . ."** Steve Johnson, "Study Weighs in on Effect of TV; Food, Obesity, Ads Target African-American Audience," *Chicago Tribune,* April 30, 2001.

page 72 **"In January 2004, the Sinai Health Institute at Mt. Sinai Hospital, in Chicago, found that 74 percent of youngsters . . ."** Grant Pick, "Slim Chance: Even a small change in habits can cut obesity down to size, but long-term successes are few," *Chicago Tribune,* April 25, 2004.

page 76 **"Unless, of course, you don't want to go home."** In-person interview with Domnique Gregory at La Rabida Children's Hospital. We had one follow-up phone conversation, and then her phone was disconnected. So additional information and quotes from her mother come from, Pick, "Slim Chance."

page 81 **"'I like girls a lot.'"** In-person and telephone interviews with Kyle Yates.

page 83 **"Researchers seriously began studying weight loss in the 1950s . . ."** Jane Fritsch, "Scientists Unmask Diet Myth Will-power," *New York Times*, October 5, 1999.

page 83 **"The behavior modification movement stems . . ."** Ibid.

page 83 **"In the 1950s, B. F. Skinner, generally considered the father of . . ."** Jody Pawel, "T.I.P.S.: Tools for Improving Parenting Skills," *Dayton Parent Magazine*, February, 1994.

page 84 **"It looked like she needed to wash her neck really bad.'"** Telephone interviews with Alicia and Clara Lay.

Chapter 3: Mothers Against Fat Kids

page 86 **"Like so many parents, Tammy Cohen and Deborah Frohlinger met through their kids."** In-person and telephone interviews, and e-mail correspondence with Tammy Cohen and Deborah Frohlinger.

page 88 **"'Letting go of weightism and accepting your child's natural build . . .'"** As quoted in "ShapeDown Parent's Guide: A Guide to Supporting Your Child." (San Anselmo, CA: Balboa Publishing, 2002), 7.

page 92 **"Currently, only about a third of all U.S. medical schools have . . ."** Telephone interview with Dr. Steven Zeisel, MD, Ph.D., professor and chair of the Department of Nutrition at the University of North Carolina, Chapel Hill.

page 92 **"An August 2003 report from the American Academy of Pediatrics . . ."** As cited in Nancy Wartik, "Rising Obesity in Children Prompts Call to Action," *New York Times,* August 26, 2003.

page 93 **"'It tells pediatricians a lot about what they should be assessing.'"** Dr. William Dietz, MD, Ph.D., director of the division of Nutrition and Physical Activity at the CDC's National Center for Chronic Disease Prevention and Health Promotions. As quoted in Wartik, "Rising Obesity."

page 95 **"Lawrence and his mother, Rhonda, have searched high and low . . ."** Telephone interview with Lawrence and Rhonda Capici.

page 96   **"'My sister is over 200 pounds . . .'"** Telephone interview with Danalee Wechsler.

page 100   **"Even experts can be baffled when it comes to their own families."** Telephone interview with Anne M. Fletcher.

page 107   **"I worked with a twelve-year-old who was upset about his weight."** Telephone interview with Ellyn Satter, MS, RD, LCSW, BCD. Other information comes from Amy Benfer, "The Lost Language of Fat," *Salon,* March 25, 2002, www.salon.com/mwt/feature/2002/03/25/fat kids/index.html.

page 110   **"No one knows unaware parents better than Christina Houghton."** In-person and telephone interview with Christina Houghton.

page 115   **"Ana was the three-year old, 120-pound girl in Albuquerque, New Mexico, who was taken . . ."** In-person interview with Adela Regino at her home. Additional information about the family and the case comes from Lisa Belkin, "Watching her Weight," *New York Times Magazine,* July 8, 2001.

page 118   **"'. . . obesity is not automatically covered by disability law . . .'"** Sandra Solovay, JD, *Tipping the Scales of Justice*: *Fighting Weight-Based Discrimination* (Amherst, NY: Prometheus Books, 2000), 146.

page 125   **"But perhaps the most famous case . . ."** I relied heavily on several different sources for information on Christina Corrigan, including Solovay, *Tipping the Scales of Justice,* pp. 13–20; Amanda Spake, "Rethinking Weight," *US News and World Report,* February 9, 2004.

page 126   **"Everyone in my family has had something with their weight . . ."** Telephone interview with Sondra Solovay.

page 126   **"Researchers at Rockefeller University . . ."** Solovay, *Tipping the Scales of Justice,* 193.

page 126   **"'Obesity is controlled by a 'powerful biological system of hormones, proteins, neurotransmitters and genes . . .'"** Dr. Louis J. Aronne, MD, FACP, director of the Comprehensive Weight Control Program at New York-Presbyterian Hospital and president of the North American Association for the Study of Obesity (NAASO), as quoted in Spake, "Rethinking Weight."

page 129   "**Alison Jeffery, a member of the research team at the Peninsula Medical School in Plymouth, England, questioned 300 seven-year-old children . . .**" Patricia Reaney, "Parents Don't See Obesity in Their Children," March 17, 2004, Reuters.

page 130   "**Can parents be sued for having an obese child?**" All the information on the court cases comes from Solovay, *Tipping the Scales of Justice*, 65–69.

page 132   "**Even when children and their parents are united in agreement . . .**" Solovay, *Tipping the Scales of Justice*, 75.

page 133   "**'I told the judge the parents are not responsible . . .'**" Telephone interview with Joanne Ikeda, co-director of the University of California, Berkeley, Center for Weight and Health.

page 133   "**'The issue of Childhood obesity is complex . . .'**" Copyright 2003 by Ellyn Satter, from www.ellynsatter.com. For more information about normal and distorted weight gain, see "Understand your child's growth," Your Child's Weight: Helping Without Harming, Kelcy Press, 2005.

Chapter 4: The Myths of Willpower and Control

page 151   "**'Teens are at the beginning of life's journey.'**" Erika Schwartz, MD, *The Teen Weight-Loss Solution* (New York: HarperCollins, 2004), 31.

page 153   "**'Exposure to fat induces a liking for fat . . .'**" E-mail correspondence with Professor John Blundell, Director of the Institute of Psychological Sciences at the University of Leeds.

page 153   "**Some researchers believe that people gain weight because they don't produce enough of the hormone PYY . . .**" Bradford McKee, "As Suburbs Grow, So Do Waistlines," *New York Times*, September 4, 2000.

page 153   "**'Overweight people are typically PYY deficient.'**" Dr. Stephen R. Bloom, professor of endocrinology, Hammersmith Hospital, Imperial College School of Medicine, London. As quoted in McKee, "As Suburbs Grow."

page 154   "'. . . placed 742 people from 213 families through a rigorous twenty-week endurance-training program.'" E-mail correspondence with Dr. Claude Bouchard, Ph.D., director of the Pennington Biomedical Research Center in Baton Rouge, Louisiana.

page 154   "'Compulsive eating is for the most part eating that's done not in response to physical hunger . . .'" Telephone interview with Dr. Sharon K. Farber, Ph.D., author of *When the Body is the Target: Self-Harm, Pain and Traumatic Attachments* (Lanham, MD: Jason Aronson, 2000).

page 156   "All forms of alcohol, cocoa, chocolate, . . .'" Kay Sheppard, *Food Addiction: The Body Knows* (Deerfield Beach, FL: HCI Books, 1993), 161.

page 156   "But new evidence seems to support the claim that you can be physiologically addicted to food . . .'" Jane Fritsch, "Scientists Unmask Diet Myth Willpower," *New York Times*, October 5, 1999.

page 156   "'There is no magical stuff inside of you called willpower . . .'" Dr. James C. Rosen, a professor of psychology at the University of Vermont, as quoted in Fristch, "Scientists Unmask."

page 157   "Drugs like fenfluramine, half of the now-banned fen-phen combination . . ." Ibid.

page 157   "In 2002, Dr. Gene-Jack Wang and his colleagues . . ." Reuters, "You May Really Be Addicted to That Chocolate Cake," April 20, 2004.

page 158   "'Chocolate is a drug of abuse in its own category.'" Dr. Louis Aronne, director of the comprehensive weight-control program at New York-Presbyterian Hospital, as quoted in Anne Underwood, "That's Why We Call It Junk Food," *Newsweek*, December 8, 2003.

page 158   "Dr. Wang has also found that merely looking at favorite foods . . ." Ibid.

page 158   "In classic addiction, the brain grows less sensitive . . ." Ibid.

page 159   "Perfectionism is a strong trait in restrictive eaters . . .'" Telephone interview with Dr. Andrew J. Hill, Ph.D., psychologist and senior lecturer in Behavioral Sciences at the University of Leeds in England.

page 159   **"In 2002, Brian Wansink, a University of Illinois nutritionist and marketing professor asked student volunteers to sit in front of bowls . . ."** Spake, "Rethinking Weight."

page 159   **"Barnard swears it's possible to retrain your taste buds . . ."** E-mail interview with Neal D. Barnard, MD, founder and president of the Physicians Committee for Responsible Medicine.

page 160   **"'Nutritional deficits are not necessary for cravings.'"** Maria Pelchat, an associate professor at the Monell Sense Center, in Philadelphia, as quoted in Sally Squires, "You Know You Crave It," *Washington Post,* June 22, 2004.

page 160   **"'The body drives them in the direction of food . . .'"** Dr. Adam Drewnowski, Ph.D., MA, Director of the Nutritional Sciences Program at the University of Washington's Center for Public Health Nutrition, in Seattle. Quoted in Squires, "You Know You Crave It."

page 160   **"'The idea that nature would leave this system to a matter of 'choice' is naïve.'"** Dr. Arthur Frank, M.D., medical director of The George Washington University Weight Management Program, in Spake, "Rethinking Weight."

Chapter 5: Honey, I Shrunk My Stomach!

page 162   **"It was Lawrence's idea to go ahead with the surgery."** Telephone interview with Lawrence Capici.

page 163   **"'It's important for kids to understand what it is that they're committing to . . .'"** Telephone interview with Dr. Louis Flancbaum, MD, Chief of Bariatric Surgery, St. Luke's-Roosevelt Hospital, New York.

page 167   **"According to the American Society of Bariatric Surgery, more than 140,000 adults underwent weight-loss surgery in 2004, up from about 16,200 in 1992."** Statistics come directly from the ASBS.

I relied on four articles for background information on bariatric surgery: Stephanie Booth, "Teenage Waistland." *Salon,* March 4, 2004, http://archive.salon.com/mwt/feature/2004/03/16/gastric bypass/index np.htm/; Ron Winslow and

Rhonda L. Rundle, "Struggling with Obesity: Obese Teens See Drastic Cure—Stomach Stapling Delivers Big Weight Loss: Should Kids Get It?" *Wall Street Journal Europe,* October 8, 2003; Emily Lambert, "Willpower-Free Dieting: Bariatric Surgery is popular, maybe a little too popular," *Forbes Magazine,* May 12, 2003; Denise Grady, "Operation for Obesity Leaves Some in Misery," *New York Times,* May 4, 2004.

page 168 **"The mortality rates, at least among adults, are relatively high . . ."** Booth, "Teenage Waistland."

page 170 **"Some suggestions indicate that the success rates are not as high . . ."** Denise Grady, "Operation for Obesity Leaves Some in Misery," *New York Times,* May 4, 2004.

page 171 **"'The whole gastric bypass universe is being driven . . .'"** Telephone interview with Dr. Henry Anhalt, MD, a pediatric endocrinologist and director of the Kids Weight Down Program at Maimonides Medical Center, Brooklyn, NY.

page 172 **"For severely obese patients, weight loss by diet . . ."** Telephone interview with Dr. Philip Schauer, MD, former director of bariatric surgery at the University of Pittsburgh Medical Center, currently a director of bariatric surgery at The Cleveland Clinic Weight Management Program.

page 172 **"In December, 2003, the FDA approved the use of the weight loss drug Xenical . . ."** Anahad O'Connor and Denise Grady, "FDA Moves to Let Drugs Treat Obese Teenagers," *New York Times,* December 13, 2003.

page 173 **"Two other prescription drugs are also on the market for kids . . ."** Sara Schaefer Munoz, "For Heavy Teens, More Options—Xenical Joins Limited Choice for Treating the Young and Obese," *Wall Street Journal,* December 17, 2003.

page 173 **"'Liposuction, a process in which surgeons dissolve fat deposits and vacuum them out . . .'"** "Liposuction Doesn't Offer Health Benefits, Study Finds," *New York Times,* June 17, 2004.

page 173 **"'What this study tells you is that losing fat itself by sucking it out . . .'"** Dr. Samuel Klein, MD, director of the Center for Human Nutrition at the Washington University School of Medicine in St. Louis, as quoted in Grady, "Liposuction Doesn't."

page 174 **"I always tell people that the operation is the first step."** In-person interview with Dr. James C. Rosser, Jr., MD chief of Minimally Invasive Surgery, Beth Israel Medical Center, Manhattan, New York.

page 176 **"Jules Hirsch, professor emeritus at Rockefeller University, in Manhattan, believes that an overabundance of fat cells . . ."** Spake, "Rethinking Weight."

page 178 **"'If we call obesity a disease, then anything that reduces . . .'"** Dr. Stephen Ball, Ph.D., State Specialist & Assistant Professor, Nutritional Sciences, College of Human Environmental Sciences, University of Missouri-Columbia as quoted in Spake, "Rethinking Weight."

page 181 **"I do believe it is sort of a grieving process.'"** Email correspondence with Wendie Pecharsky.

page 181 **"'My whole life I was overweight . . .'"** In-person interview with Tricia Winfield.

page 183 **"Joshua Gee, who lives outside Erie, Pennsylvania, was seventeen . . ."** Telephone interview with Joshua and Michelle Gee, and Ken Pulos. Other information comes from Cristina Rouvalis, "More Than Meets the Eye and Erie Teen Becomes the Third Generation of His Family to Choose Gastric Bypass as an Escape from Obesity," *Pittsburgh Post-Gazette*, October 12, 2003.

Chapter 6: Size Acceptance: Fat or Fiction?

page 186 **"Diets, she believes, fail 95 percent of the time . . ."** Telephone interview with Joanne Ikeda.

page 186 **"From 2000 to 2001, Ikeda and her colleagues surveyed 149 obese women . . ."** From Joanne Ikeda, "Self-reported dieting experiences of women with body mass indexes of 30 or more," *Journal of American Dietetic Association*, 104(6), 972–975.

page 187 **"'There is some thought that continuous dieting . . .'"** Dr. Julie Miller Jones, Ph.D., professor of nutrition and food science at the College of St. Catherine. Ibid.

page 188 **"Burgard is not anti-exercise but she is vehemently anti-weight loss . . ."** Telephone interview with Dr. Debby Burgard,

Ph.D., clinical psychologist in Los Altos, California, and the founder of Body Positive (www.bodypositive.com).

page 189   **"That's what happened six years ago, after former New England Journal of Medicine editor . . ."** There have been many articles written about this topic, including "Weight vs. Fitness: the Debate Continues," in the *Star Banner*, June 27,2004. http://64.233.161.104/search?q=cache:APoGlfSdyicJ: www.starbanner.com/apps/pbcs.dll/article%3FAID%3D/2004 0627/NEWS/206270351/1017/FEATURES04%26template%3 Dprintart+%22Jerome+Kassirer%22++%22limited,+fragmentary +and+often+ambiguous.%22++&hl=en.

page 190   **"Contrary to almost everything you have heard . . ."** Professor Paul Campos of the University of Colorado School of Law, as quoted in Dinitia Smith, "Demonizing Fat in the War on Weight," *New York Times,* May 1, 2004.

page 190   **"If you take fat people who have all these health problems . . ."** Glenn A. Gaesser, Ph.D., professor of exercise physiology at the University of Virginia, as quoted in "Can Being Fit Outweigh Fat? It's Possible to Be Obese and Healthy, Experts Say." *Washington Post*, November 26, 2004. Also e-mail correspondence with Gaesser.

page 190   **"Losing ten or fifteen pounds might be enough . . ."** Daniel Q. Haney, "Losing a Few Pounds May Help the Obese," *Associated Press*, June 1, 2004.

page 190   **"Houston cardiologist Christie Ballantyne watched patients . . ."** Ibid.

page 190   **"'Our knowledge of weight and weight-related disorders . . .'"** Telephone interview with Dr. Henry Anhalt.

page 192   **"'It's cruel and criminal that the obesity mafia . . .'"** Telephone interview with Marilyn Wann. She mentioned Kelly Yeomans, Samuel Graham, and Brian Head to me, and I then researched them on the web at www.seafattle.org.

page 194   **"Not that progress hasn't been made on the body-love front . . ."** Mary DuenwaL.D., "One Size Definitely Does Not Fit All," *New York Times*, June 22, 2003. Also Ginia Bellafante, "Young and Chubby: What's heavy about that?" *New York Times,* January 26, 2003.

page 196   **"Fat activists, of course, don't see it that way . . ."** Telephone interview with Pat Lyons.

page 197   **"'I don't really watch too much what other mothers are doing . . .'"** Telephone interview with Beth and Shandra Swilling.

page 199   **"'There's a lot of weight on her . . .'"** Telephone interview with Alison Solomon.

page 200   **"Setnick takes a non-diet approach to weight loss . . ."** Telephone interview with Jessica Setnick, MS, RD, LD.

Chapter 7: Inner Fat Camp

page 207   **"'If anyone believes that one skill . . .'"** Telephone interview with Professor Paul Gately, Ph.D., director of the children's weight loss program at Leeds Metropolitan University in England.

page 209   **"'You've got to make small steps, and appreciate that you can't have . . .'"** Telephone interview with Dr. Henry Anhalt.

page 210   **"'You have to want to be thin . . .'"** Telephone interview with Anne M. Fletcher.

page 211   **"As we listened to our participants, we became aware . . .'"** Email correspondence with Dr. James O. Prochaska, Ph.D., director of the Cancer Prevention Research Center and professor of Clinical and Health Psychology at the University of Rhode Island.

page 213   **"Let go of trying to change weight . . .'"** These acceptance tenets come from Debby Burgard's Web site, www.body positive.com/childwt.htm, and are gratefully reprinted with her permission.

page 213   **"'You're never too young . . .'"** In-person interview with Danielle Webber (not her real name).

page 214   **"When my daughter wants to eat, I'll say . . . '"** Telephone interview with Bonnie Werth and Alexis Werth Mason.

page 216   **"'six thousand dollars is a lot of money . . .'"** Telephone interview with Shawn and Zach Lowe.

select bibliography

Brownell, Kelly D., Ph.D., and Katherine Battle Horgen. *Food Fight: The Inside Story of the Food Industry, America's Obesity Crisis, and What We Can Do About It.* (New York: McGraw-Hill, 2003).

Campos, Paul. *The Obesity Myth: Why America's Obsession Is Hazardous to Your Health.* (New York: Gotham Books, 2004).

Crister, Greg. *Fat Land: How Americans Became the Fattest People in the World.* (Boston: Houghton Mifflin, 2003).

Emme. *True Beauty: Positive Attitudes and Practical Tips from the World's Leading Plus-Size Model.* (New York: Putnam Publishing Group, 1997).

Emme. *Life's Little Emergencies: Everyday Rescue for Beauty, Fashion, Relationships and Life.* (New York: St. Martin's Press, 2003).

Fumento, Michael. *The Fat of the Land: Our Health Crisis and How Overweight Americans Can Help Themselves.* (New York: Viking, 1998).

Flancbaum, Louis, MD. *The Doctor's Guide to Weight Loss Surgery: How to Make the Decisions that Could Save Your Life.* (New York: Bantam Books, 2003).

Fletcher, Anne. *Thin for Life: 10 Keys to Success from People Who Have Lost Weight and Kept It Off.* (Boston: Houghton Mifflin, 2003).

Kirschenbaum, Daniel S., Ph.D., *The 9 Truths about Weight Loss: The No-Tricks, No Nonsense Plan for Lifelong Weight Control.* (New York: Owl Books, 2001).

McGraw, Jay. *The Ultimate Weight Solution for Teens: The 7 Keys to Weight Freedom.* (New York: Free Press, 2003).

Nichter, Mimi. *Fat Talk: What Girls and Their Parents Say about Dieting.* (Boston: Harvard College, 2000).

Rimm, Sylvia B. *Rescuing the Emotional Lives of Overweight Children.* (New York: Rodale, St. Martin's Press, 2004).

Schlosser, Eric. *Fast Food Nation: The Dark Side of the All-American Meal.* (New York: Perennial, 2002).

Schwartz, Erika, MD. *The Teen-Weight-Loss Solution: The Safe and Effective Path to Health and Self-Confidence.* (New York: William Morrow, 2004).

Shell, Ellen Ruppel. *The Hungry Gene: The Inside Story of the Obesity Industry.* (New York: Grove Press, 2002).

Solovay, Sandra, JD. *Tipping the Scales of Justice: Fighting Weight-Based Discrimination.* (Amherst, NY: Prometheus Books, 2000).

Sothern, Melinda, S., and T. Kristian von Almen. *Trim Kids: The Proven 12-Week Plan That Has Helped Thousands of Children Achieve a Healthier Weight.* (New York: HarperResource, 2003).

Wann, Marilyn. *Fat! SO? Because You Don't Have to Apologize for Your Size.* (Berkeley, CA: Ten Speed Press, 1999).

index

PublicAffairs is a publishing house founded in 1997. It is a tribute to the standards, values, and flair of three persons who have served as mentors to countless reporters, writers, editors, and book people of all kinds, including me.

I. F. Stone, proprietor of *I. F. Stone's Weekly,* combined a commitment to the First Amendment with entrepreneurial zeal and reporting skill and became one of the great independent journalists in American history. At the age of eighty, Izzy published *The Trial of Socrates,* which was a national bestseller. He wrote the book after he taught himself ancient Greek.

Benjamin C. Bradlee was for nearly thirty years the charismatic editorial leader of *The Washington Post.* It was Ben who gave the *Post* the range and courage to pursue such historic issues as Watergate. He supported his reporters with a tenacity that made them fearless, and it is no accident that so many became authors of influential, best-selling books.

Robert L. Bernstein, the chief executive of Random House for more than a quarter century, guided one of the nation's premier publishing houses. Bob was personally responsible for many books of political dissent and argument that challenged tyranny around the globe. He is also the founder and was the longtime chair of Human Rights Watch, one of the most respected human rights organizations in the world.

· · ·

For fifty years, the banner of Public Affairs Press was carried by its owner, Morris B. Schnapper, who published Gandhi, Nasser, Toynbee, Truman, and about 1,500 other authors. In 1983 Schnapper was described by *The Washington Post* as "a redoubtable gadfly." His legacy will endure in the books to come.

Peter Osnos, *Publisher*